No Gluten, No Problem, Cookbook

The Ultimate Gluten-Free Recipe Collection for Every Home Cook

By: Owen Davis

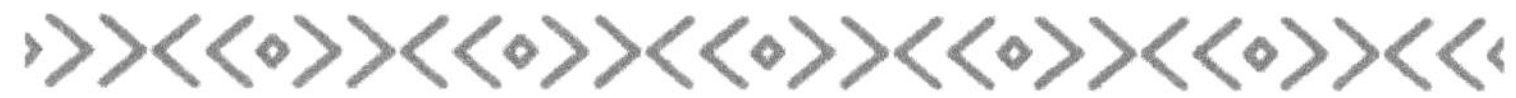

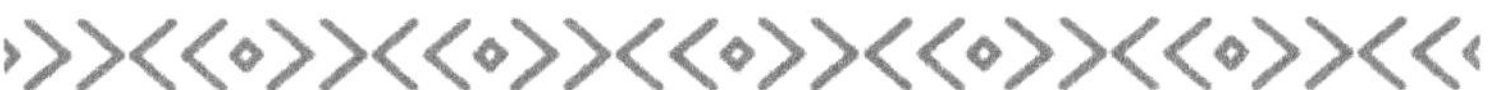

Table of Contents

Introduction 5

1. Quinoa and Roasted Vegetable Salad with Lemon Vinaigrette..............................6

2. Zucchini Noodles with Pesto and Cherry Tomatoes 9

3. Chickpea Flour Pancakes with Avocado and Salsa................................12

4. Butternut Squash and Sage Risotto 15

5. Cauliflower Pizza Crust with Fresh Mozzarella and Basil 18

6. Sweet Potato and Black Bean Tacos with Cilantro-Lime Slaw............................21

7. Spinach and Feta Stuffed Mushrooms..24

8. Thai-inspired Coconut Curry with Tofu and Vegetables................................27

9. Almond-Crusted Baked Chicken Tenders 30

10. Mediterranean Grilled Eggplant Rolls with Hummus 33

11. Creamy Broccoli and Cheddar Soup 36

12. Herbed Quinoa-Stuffed Bell Peppers 39

13. Gluten-Free Blueberry Muffins with Streusel Topping................................42

14. Chocolate Avocado Mousse with Berries 45

15. Spaghetti Squash Primavera with Garlic-Herb Sauce 47

16. Roasted Beet and Goat Cheese Salad with Balsamic Glaze 50

17. Oven-baked Garlic Parmesan Fries 53

18. Mexican Cauliflower Rice Bowl with Guacamole and Salsa 56

19. Apple Cinnamon Quinoa Porridge 59

20. Caprese Salad Skewers with Balsamic Reduction 62

21. Crispy Baked Fish Tacos with Cabbage Slaw.. 64

22. Caramelized Onion and Goat Cheese Frittata 67

23. Pomegranate and Spinach Salad with Honey Mustard Dressing 70

24. Baked Portobello Mushrooms with Quinoa Stuffing 73

25. Chocolate Peanut Butter Energy Bites.. 76

26. Roasted Vegetable Frittata with Fresh Herbs.. 78

27. Blackened Shrimp with Mango-Avocado Salsa.. 81

28. Lemon Poppy Seed Almond Flour Pancakes 84

29. Roasted Red Pepper and Tomato Soup... 87

30. Berry Parfait with Greek Yogurt and Granola 90

Conclusion 92

Appendices 93

Introduction

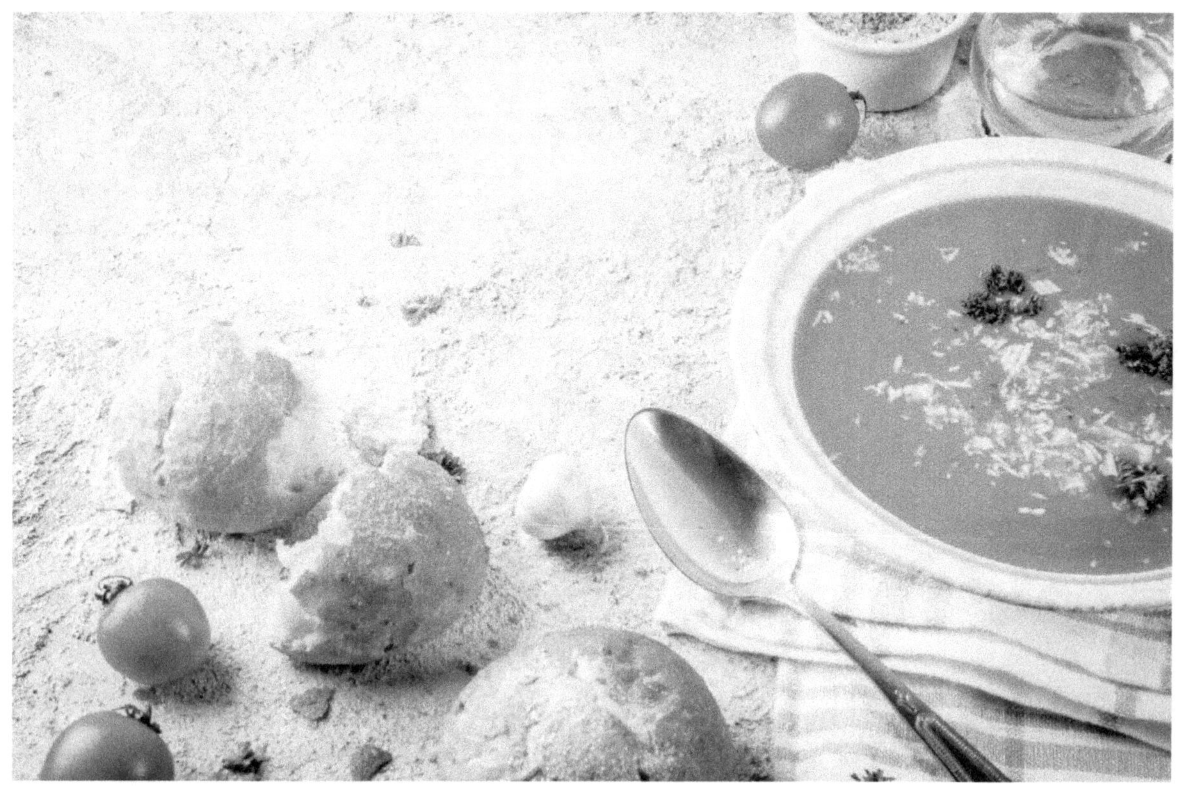

Welcome to a world where gluten-free cooking knows no bounds. As a passionate cook and lover of food, I've delved into the realm of gluten-free cooking with enthusiasm and creativity. This cookbook is a reflection of my exploration, featuring a curated collection of 30 recipes that will captivate your taste buds and nourish your body.

Each dish has been meticulously designed to showcase the incredible potential of gluten-free ingredients. Whether you're a seasoned gluten-free advocate or simply seeking flavorful alternatives, this cookbook is a gateway to a world of possibilities.

1. Quinoa and Roasted Vegetable Salad with Lemon Vinaigrette

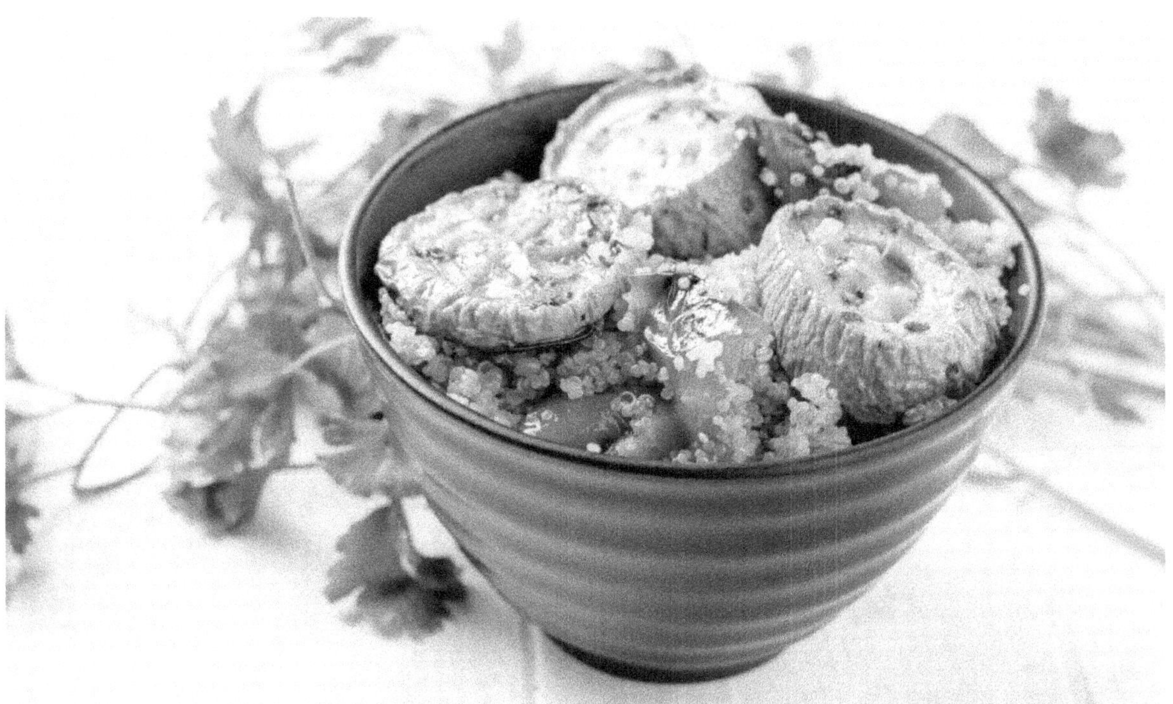

As someone who's always seeking vibrant and nutritious meals, my Quinoa and Roasted Vegetable Salad with Lemon Vinaigrette has become a staple in my kitchen. This dish is a celebration of colors, flavors, and textures that dance harmoniously on the palate. The nutty quinoa paired with the sweetness of roasted vegetables is a symphony of goodness. With every bite, I'm reminded that eating gluten-free doesn't mean compromising on taste or satisfaction. Crafting this salad is like painting a canvas of culinary delight—a creation that nourishes both body and soul.

Serving Size: 4 servings

Preparation Time: 15 minutes

Cooking Time: 25 minutes

Ingredients:

- Quinoa rinsed and drained (1 cup)
- Mixed vegetables- bell peppers, zucchini, cherry tomatoes, red onion, diced (2 cups)
- Olive oil (2 tablespoons)
- Salt and pepper, to taste
- Fresh parsley, chopped (1/4 cup)
- Feta cheese, crumbled (optional) (1/4 cup)
- Lemon Vinaigrette:
- Extra virgin olive oil (1/4 cup)
- Fresh lemon juice (2 tablespoons)
- Dijon mustard (1 teaspoon)
- Garlic, minced (1 clove)
- Salt and pepper, to taste

Instructions:

In a medium saucepan, bring 2 cups of water to a boil. Add the rinsed quinoa and a pinch of salt. Reduce the heat to low, cover, and then let it simmer for 15 minutes, or until the quinoa is fluffy and the water is absorbed. Remove from heat and fluff with a fork.

Preheat your oven to 400°F (200°C). Toss the diced mixed vegetables with olive oil, salt, and pepper. Spread them on a baking sheet and roast for about 20-25 minutes, or until they're tender and slightly caramelized.

In a small bowl, whisk together the extra virgin olive oil, Dijon mustard, fresh lemon juice, minced garlic, salt, and pepper. This zesty vinaigrette is the heart of the dish.

In a large bowl, combine the cooked quinoa and roasted vegetables. Drizzle the lemon vinaigrette over the mixture. Gently toss to coat everything in the vibrant flavors.

Sprinkle chopped fresh parsley over the salad. The parsley adds a burst of color and freshness. If desired, crumble feta cheese over the top. The creamy cheese is a delightful contrast to the hearty quinoa and vegetables. Portion the Quinoa and Roasted Vegetable Salad into bowls or on plates.

2. Zucchini Noodles with Pesto and Cherry Tomatoes

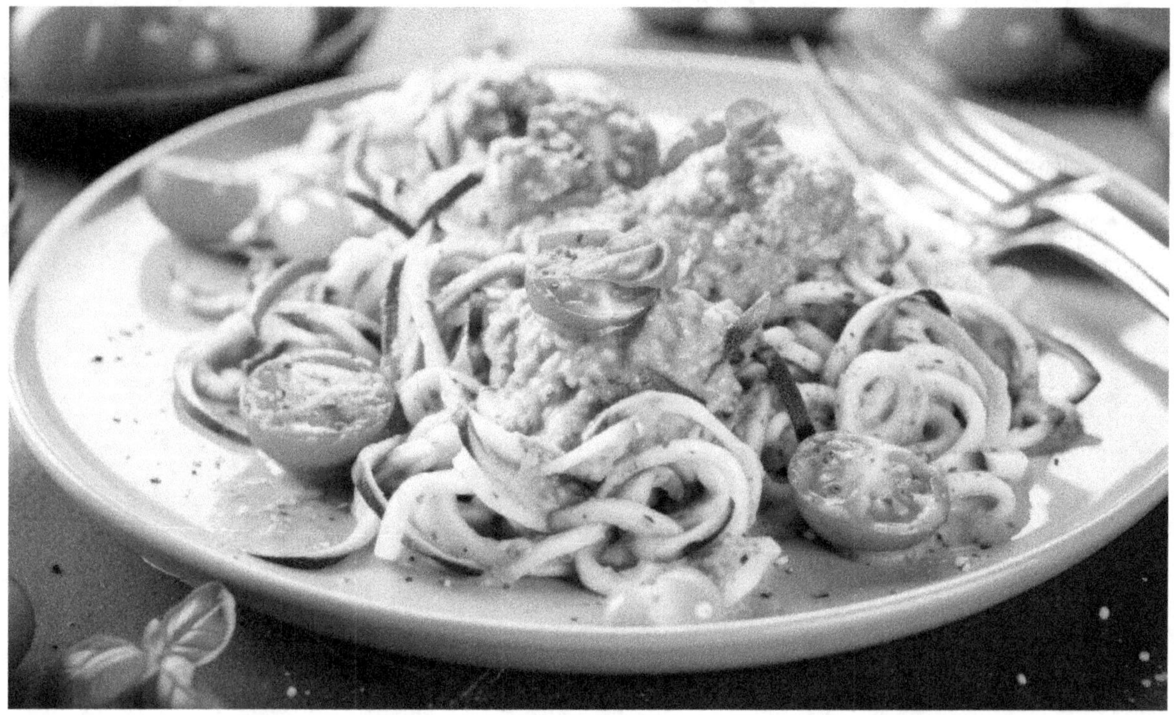

There's a certain kind of magic that happens when you transform humble zucchinis into delicate, ribbon-like noodles. My Zucchini Noodles with Pesto and Cherry Tomatoes is a celebration of this magic—a dish that bursts with vibrant colors and flavors that awaken the senses. As someone who cherishes both healthful and delightful meals, this recipe has earned a special place in my kitchen. Crafting this dish is like creating a work of art—a culinary masterpiece that brings joy to every forkful.

Serving Size: 2 servings

Preparation Time: 15 minutes

Cooking Time: 5 minutes

Ingredients:

- Medium zucchinis, spiralized into noodles (2)
- Cherry tomatoes, halved (1 cup)
- Pesto sauce (store-bought or homemade) (1/4 cup)
- Pine nuts, toasted (2 tablespoons)
- Grated Parmesan cheese, for garnish (optional)
- Fresh basil leaves, for garnish
- Salt and pepper, to taste
- Olive oil, for sautéing

Instructions:

Use a spiralizer to turn the zucchini into noodles. If you don't have a spiralizer, you can also use a julienne peeler to create thin strips.

In a dry skillet over medium heat, toast the pine nuts until they're golden and fragrant. Keep a close eye on them, as they can quickly go from toasted to burnt.

In the same skillet, add a drizzle of olive oil over medium heat. Add the zucchini noodles and sauté them for about 2-3 minutes, or until they're just tender. Be careful not to overcook, as zucchini noodles can become mushy.

Toss in the halved cherry tomatoes and sauté for an additional 1-2 minutes, just until they're slightly softened.

Lower the heat and add the pesto sauce to the skillet. Gently toss the zucchini noodles and cherry tomatoes in the pesto until they're well coated.

Season with salt and pepper to taste. The pesto is already flavorful, so a little goes a long way. Divide the Zucchini Noodles with Pesto and Cherry Tomatoes between serving plates. Sprinkle toasted pine nuts over the top, along with grated Parmesan cheese if desired.

3. Chickpea Flour Pancakes with Avocado and Salsa

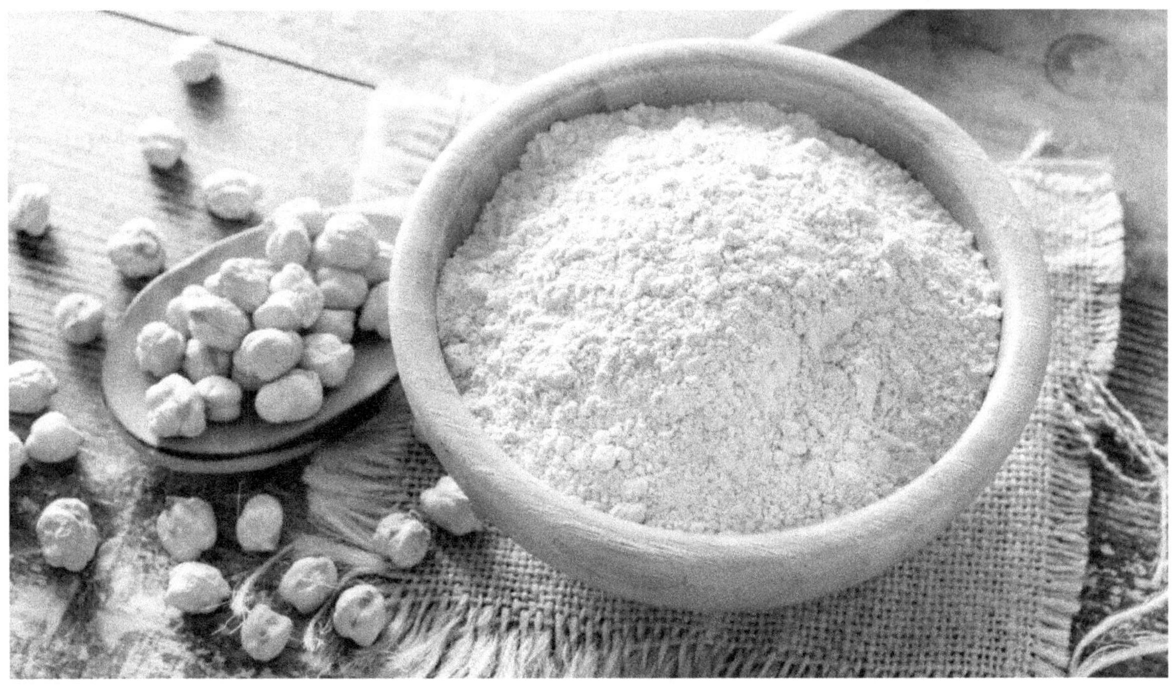

In the realm of gluten-free cooking, creativity knows no bounds. That's why my Chickpea Flour Pancakes with Avocado and Salsa have become a staple in my culinary repertoire. These pancakes are a delightful twist on the classic, infused with the goodness of chickpea flour—a versatile ingredient that's both nutritious and flavorful. Each bite is a symphony of textures and tastes that leave me feeling both satisfied and invigorated. Preparing this dish is like crafting a masterpiece—a medley of ingredients that come together in perfect harmony.

Serving Size: 2 servings

Preparation Time: 10 minutes

Cooking Time: 15 minutes

Ingredients: For the Chickpea Flour Pancakes:

- Chickpea flour (1 cup)

- Baking powder (1/2 teaspoon)

- Ground turmeric (optional, for color) (1/4 teaspoon)

- Salt and pepper, to taste

- Water (3/4 cup)

- Olive oil (2 tablespoons)

- For the Avocado and Salsa Topping:

- Avocado, sliced (1)

- Fresh salsa (store-bought or homemade) (1/2 cup)

- Fresh cilantro leaves, for garnish

- Lime wedges, for serving

Instructions:

In a mixing bowl, whisk together the chickpea flour, baking powder, ground turmeric (if using), salt, and pepper. Gradually add water while whisking to form a smooth batter. Let the batter sit for about 5 minutes to allow the chickpea flour to absorb the liquid.

Heat a non-stick skillet over medium heat. Drizzle a bit of olive oil and spread it evenly. Pour a ladleful of the chickpea flour batter onto the skillet to form a pancake. Cook for about 2-3 minutes on each side, until golden brown and cooked through. Repeat with the remaining batter.

Place the cooked chickpea flour pancakes on serving plates. Layer the sliced avocado on top of the pancakes.

Spoon a generous amount of fresh salsa over the avocado. The vibrant colors are a visual feast.

Sprinkle fresh cilantro leaves over the top. The aromatic herb adds a burst of freshness.

Serve the Chickpea Flour Pancakes with Avocado and Salsa with lime wedges on the side. A squeeze of lime adds a zesty finish.

4. Butternut Squash and Sage Risotto

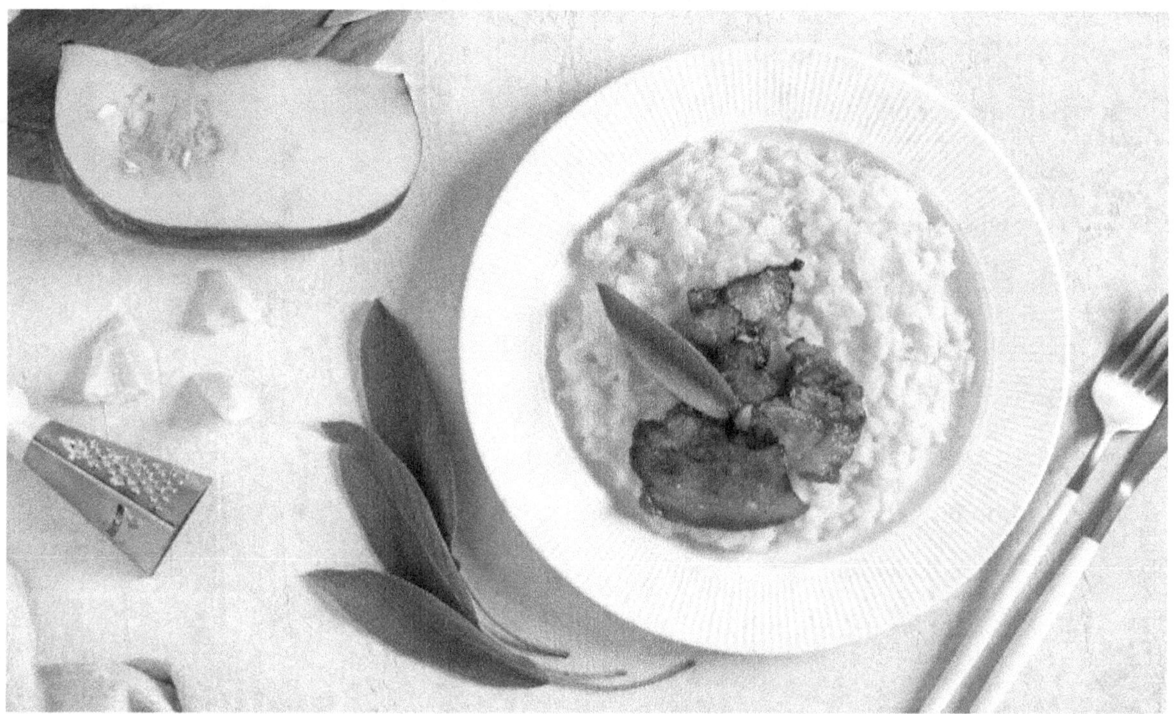

There's something truly magical about the fusion of creamy risotto with the earthy sweetness of butternut squash and the aromatic charm of sage. My Butternut Squash and Sage Risotto is a symphony of flavors that dances on the taste buds—a dish that captures the essence of comfort and sophistication. As someone who finds joy in gluten-free cooking, this recipe has earned a special place in my heart. Preparing this risotto is like crafting a culinary masterpiece—a medley of ingredients that come together to create a sensation of warmth and indulgence.

Serving Size: 4 servings

Preparation Time: 10 minutes

Cooking Time: 30 minutes

Ingredients:

- Small butternut squash, peeled, seeded, and diced (1)
- Olive oil (2 tablespoons)
- Salt and pepper, to taste
- Arborio rice (1 cup)
- Dry white wine (optional) (1/2 cup)
- Vegetable broth, warmed (4 cups)
- Grated Parmesan cheese (1/2 cup)
- Butter (2 tablespoons)
- Fresh sage leaves, chopped (1 tablespoon)
- Additional sage leaves, for garnish

Instructions:

Preheat your oven to 400°F (200°C). Toss the diced butternut squash with olive oil, salt, and pepper. Spread them on a baking sheet and roast for about 20-25 minutes, or until they're tender and slightly caramelized. Set aside.

In a large skillet or pan, heat a drizzle of olive oil over medium heat. Add the Arborio rice and toast it for about 2 minutes until the edges turn translucent.

Pour in the dry white wine and let it simmer until it's mostly absorbed by the rice. This step adds a layer of depth to the risotto.

Begin adding warm vegetable broth to the rice, one ladleful at a time. Allow the broth to be absorbed before adding more. Stir constantly to encourage the creamy texture to develop.

Continue adding broth and stirring until the rice is tender and creamy. This should take around 20-25 minutes. The risotto should have a slightly al dente texture.

Gently fold in the roasted butternut squash cubes, allowing them to mingle with the velvety rice.

Stir in the chopped fresh sage leaves, grated Parmesan cheese, and butter. The sage adds an aromatic note that beautifully complements the sweetness of the squash.

Season with salt and pepper to taste. The dish should be rich and harmonious.

5. Cauliflower Pizza Crust with Fresh Mozzarella and Basil

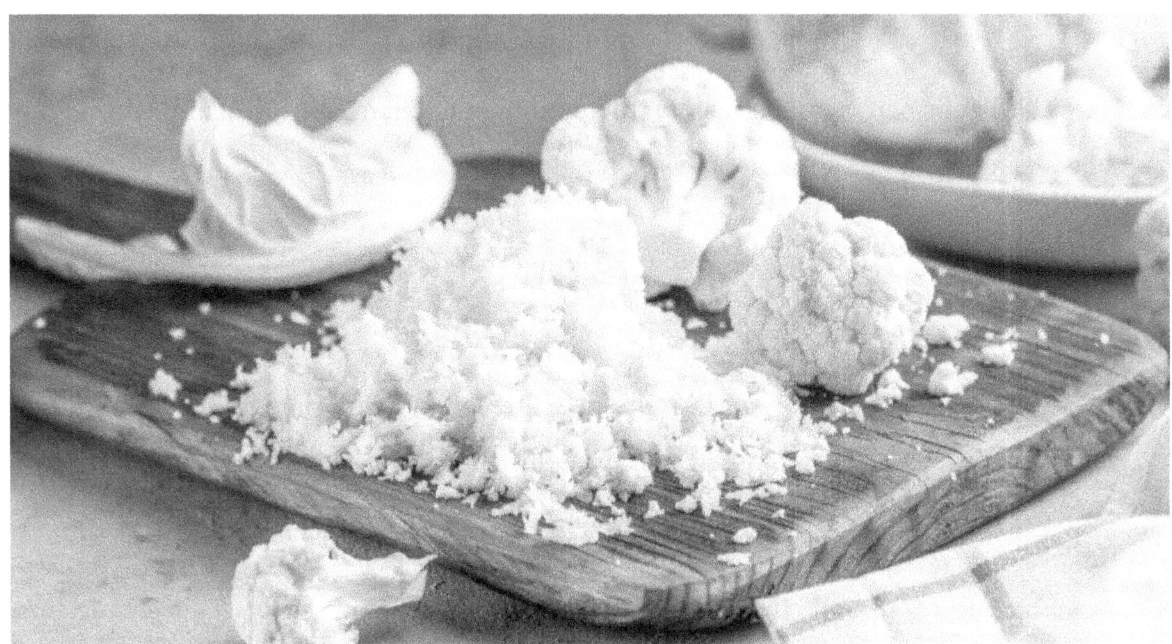

Amid the world of gluten-free cooking, few things rival the sheer delight of biting into a crisp, flavorful pizza. My Cauliflower Pizza Crust with Fresh Mozzarella and Basil is a revelation—an ode to both health-conscious eating and the pursuit of culinary satisfaction. Crafting this pizza crust is like painting on a canvas of wholesome ingredients—a creation that bursts with flavors, textures, and colors that ignite the senses. As a lover of gluten-free delights, this recipe has found a permanent spot in my kitchen.

Serving Size: 2 servings

Preparation Time: 20 minutes

Cooking Time: 25 minutes

Ingredients: For the Cauliflower Crust:

- Small head cauliflower, florets separated (1)
- Grated Parmesan cheese (1/2 cup)
- Egg (1)
- Dried oregano (1 teaspoon)
- Garlic powder (1/2 teaspoon)
- Salt and pepper, to taste

For the Pizza Toppings:

- Tomato sauce (store-bought or homemade) (1/2 cup)
- Fresh mozzarella cheese, sliced (1 1/2 cups)
- Fresh basil leaves, for topping
- Crushed red pepper flakes, for optional heat

Instructions:

Preheat your oven to 400°F (200°C). Steam or microwave the cauliflower florets until they're tender. Allow them to cool slightly before proceeding.

Using a food processor or a box grater, rice the steamed cauliflower until it resembles fine grains.

Place the riced cauliflower in a clean kitchen towel or cheesecloth. Squeeze out as much moisture as possible. This step is essential for achieving a crisp crust.

In a mixing bowl, combine the squeezed cauliflower, grated Parmesan cheese, egg, dried oregano, garlic powder, salt, and pepper. Mix until everything is well combined.

Line a baking sheet with parchment paper. Place the cauliflower mixture onto the parchment paper and shape it into a round pizza crust, about 1/4-inch thick.

Bake the cauliflower crust in the preheated oven for about 15 minutes, or until it's firm and golden.

Spread tomato sauce evenly over the pre-baked crust. Top with slices of fresh mozzarella cheese.

Place the pizza back in the oven and bake for an additional 10 minutes, or until the cheese is melted and bubbly.

Remove the pizza from the oven and top with fresh basil leaves. Their aromatic scent enhances the experience.

For those who enjoy a bit of heat, sprinkle crushed red pepper flakes over the pizza. Carefully slice the Cauliflower Pizza Crust with Fresh Mozzarella and Basil. Each bite is a harmonious blend of textures and flavors.

6. Sweet Potato and Black Bean Tacos with Cilantro-Lime Slaw

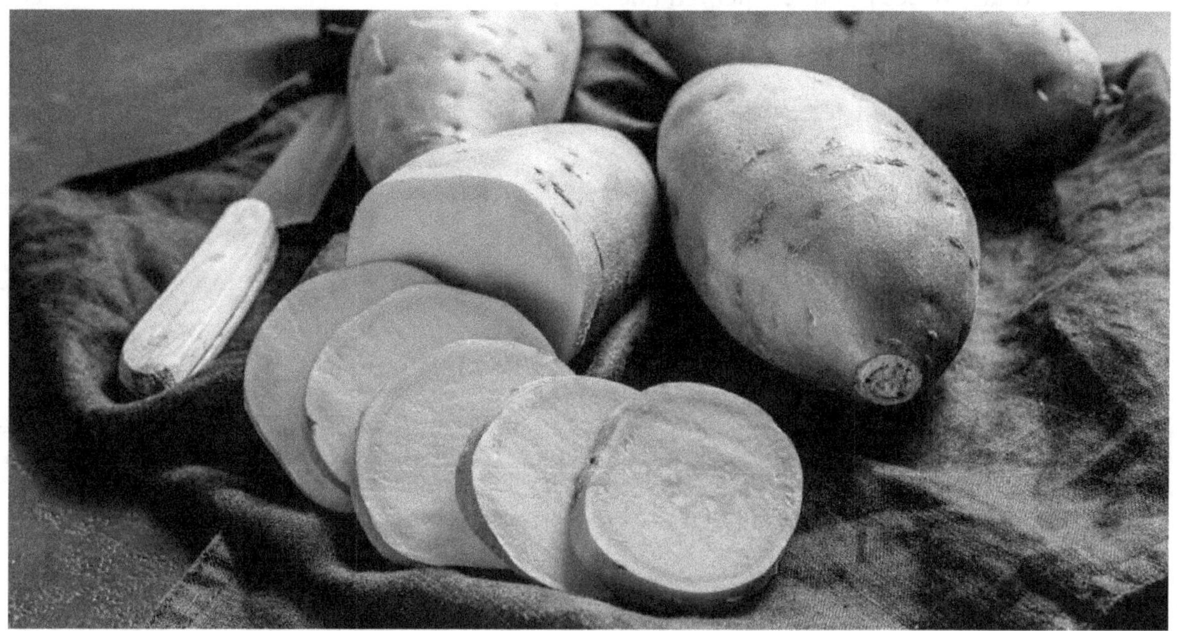

In the realm of gluten-free cuisine, the world of flavors is limitless, and my Sweet Potato and Black Bean Tacos with Cilantro-Lime Slaw are a testament to this. The fusion of tender sweet potatoes, hearty black beans, and the vibrant zing of cilantro-lime slaw is a harmonious symphony that takes taco night to a whole new level. As someone who appreciates the art of crafting satisfying meals, this recipe has become a star in my kitchen. Preparing these tacos is like composing a melody of ingredients that resonate with every bite.

Serving Size: 2 servings

Preparation Time: 15 minutes

Cooking Time: 25 minutes

Ingredients: For the Sweet Potato and Black Bean Filling:

- Medium sweet potatoes, peeled and diced (2)
- Olive oil (1 tablespoon)
- Ground cumin (1 teaspoon)
- Chili powder (1 teaspoon)
- Salt and pepper, to taste
- Black beans, drained and rinsed (1 can)

For the Cilantro-Lime Slaw:

- Shredded cabbage or coleslaw mix (1 cup)
- Fresh cilantro leaves, chopped (1/4 cup)
- Juice of 1 lime
- Greek yogurt (or mayonnaise for creamier slaw) (2 tablespoons)
- Salt and pepper, to taste

For Assembling:

- Small gluten-free corn tortillas (6)
- Crumbled feta cheese, for topping
- Fresh lime wedges, for serving

Instructions:

Preheat your oven to 400°F (200°C). Toss the diced sweet potatoes with olive oil, ground cumin, chili powder, salt, and pepper. Spread them on a baking sheet and roast for about 20-25 minutes, or until they're tender and slightly caramelized. Set aside.

In a bowl, combine the shredded cabbage, chopped cilantro, lime juice, and Greek yogurt. Mix well until the slaw is coated in the creamy dressing. Season with salt and pepper to taste.

In a saucepan, warm the black beans over medium heat. Season with a pinch of cumin, chili powder, salt, and pepper. Stir occasionally until the beans are heated through.

Heat the gluten-free corn tortillas in a dry skillet over medium heat for about 15-20 seconds on each side. This step makes them pliable and ready for filling.

On each warmed tortilla, layer a generous spoonful of the roasted sweet potatoes and warm black beans. Top with a scoop of the zesty cilantro-lime slaw.

Sprinkle crumbled feta cheese over the filling. The salty tanginess complements the other flavors beautifully.

Squeeze fresh lime juice over the tacos for a burst of zesty freshness.

Gently fold the tortillas to encase the flavorful fillings. Every bite is a dance of textures and tastes.

7. Spinach and Feta Stuffed Mushrooms

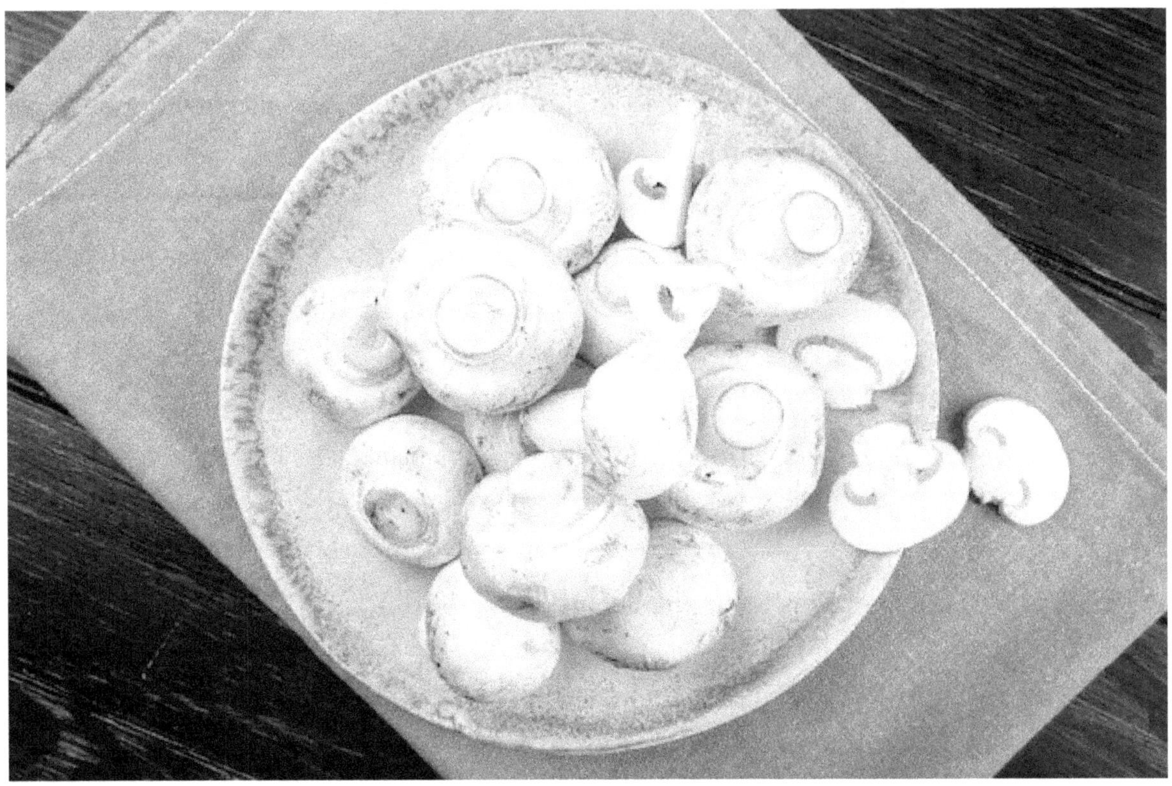

When it comes to gluten-free indulgence, my Spinach and Feta Stuffed Mushrooms are a bite-sized delight that never fails to impress. The marriage of earthy mushrooms with the vibrant flavors of spinach and tangy feta is a celebration of textures and tastes that make every nibble sensational. As someone who savors the art of crafting appetizers, this recipe holds a special place in my collection. Preparing these stuffed mushrooms is like sculpting a masterpiece—a balance of ingredients that results in pure satisfaction.

Serving Size: 4 servings (approximately 16 stuffed mushrooms)

Preparation Time: 15 minutes

Cooking Time: 25 minutes

Ingredients:

- Medium-sized white button mushrooms (16)
- Olive oil (1 tablespoon)
- Garlic, minced (2 cloves)
- Fresh spinach leaves, chopped (2 cups)
- Crumbled feta cheese (1/2 cup)
- Grated Parmesan cheese (1/4 cup)
- Salt and pepper, to taste
- Fresh parsley leaves, for garnish

Instructions:

Preheat your oven to 375°F (190°C). Gently wipe the mushrooms clean with a damp cloth. Carefully remove the stems and set them aside. Arrange the mushroom caps on a baking sheet.

In a skillet, heat olive oil over medium heat. Add minced garlic and sauté for about 1 minute until fragrant. Add the chopped spinach and cook until wilted, approximately 2-3 minutes.

In a mixing bowl, combine the sautéed spinach, crumbled feta cheese, grated Parmesan cheese, salt, and pepper. Mix well to create a flavorful stuffing.

Take each mushroom cap and fill it generously with the spinach and cheese mixture, pressing down slightly to pack the filling.

Place the stuffed mushrooms in the preheated oven and bake for about 15-20 minutes, or until the mushrooms are tender and the cheese is melted and golden.

Once out of the oven, sprinkle fresh parsley leaves over the stuffed mushrooms. The vibrant green adds a burst of color and freshness.

Arrange the Spinach and Feta Stuffed Mushrooms on a serving platter. These bite-sized gems are ready to be enjoyed.

8. Thai-inspired Coconut Curry with Tofu and Vegetables

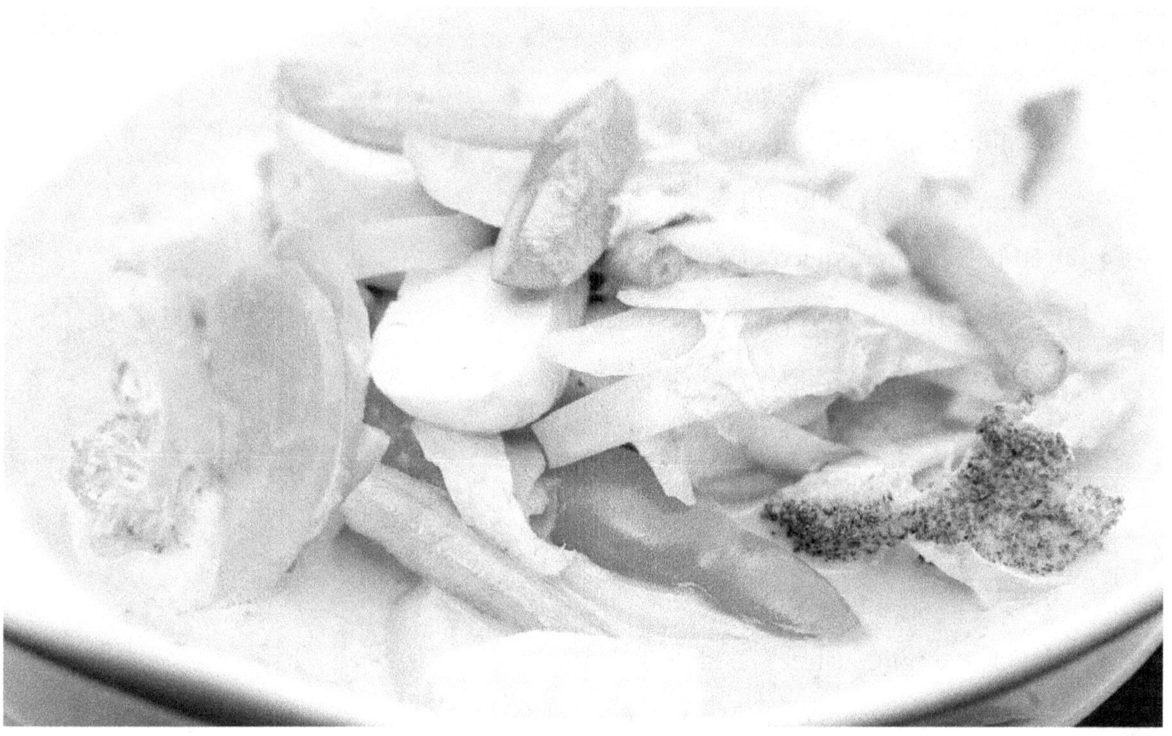

Embarking on a gluten-free culinary journey, my Thai-inspired coconut Curry with Tofu and Vegetables is a symphony of exotic flavors that whisk me away to the bustling streets of Thailand. The delicate dance of creamy coconut milk, aromatic spices, tender tofu, and vibrant vegetables creates a harmony that enchants the palate. As someone who revels in the art of global cuisine, this recipe stands as a testament to the incredible variety that gluten-free cooking has to offer. Preparing this curry is like weaving a tapestry of tastes that transport me to distant lands.

Serving Size: 4 servings

Preparation Time: 15 minutes

Cooking Time: 25 minutes

Ingredients:

- Coconut oil (1 tablespoon)
- Small onion, thinly sliced ()1
- Garlic, minced (2 cloves)
- Red bell pepper, sliced (1)
- Broccoli florets (1 cup)
- Carrots, sliced (1 cup)
- Firm tofu, cubed (1 block)
- Thai red curry paste (2 tablespoons)
- Coconut milk (1 can)
- Vegetable broth (1 cup)
- Soy sauce (gluten-free) (2 tablespoons)
- Brown sugar or coconut sugar (1 tablespoon)
- Fresh lime juice (1 tablespoon)
- Salt and pepper, to taste
- Fresh cilantro leaves, for garnish

Instructions:

In a large skillet or wok, heat coconut oil over medium heat. Add sliced onion and sauté for about 2-3 minutes until softened and slightly golden. Stir in minced garlic and cook for an additional 30 seconds.

Add the cubed tofu to the skillet and cook until it's lightly browned on all sides, about 5-7 minutes. Remove the tofu from the skillet and set it aside.

In the same skillet, add the sliced red bell pepper, broccoli florets, and sliced carrots. Sauté for about 5 minutes until the vegetables are slightly tender.

Stir in the Thai red curry paste and cook for 1-2 minutes, allowing the spices to bloom and infuse into the vegetables.

Pour in the coconut milk and vegetable broth. Bring the mixture to a gentle simmer.

Add soy sauce, brown sugar (or coconut sugar), and fresh lime juice to the curry. These elements balance the flavors beautifully.

Return the cooked tofu to the skillet, allowing it to soak up the fragrant curry sauce.

Season the curry with salt and pepper to taste. Give it a final stir, ensuring that all the ingredients are well-coated in the creamy sauce.

Ladle the Thai-inspired coconut Curry with Tofu and Vegetables into bowls. Garnish with fresh cilantro leaves for a burst of freshness.

9. Almond-Crusted Baked Chicken Tenders

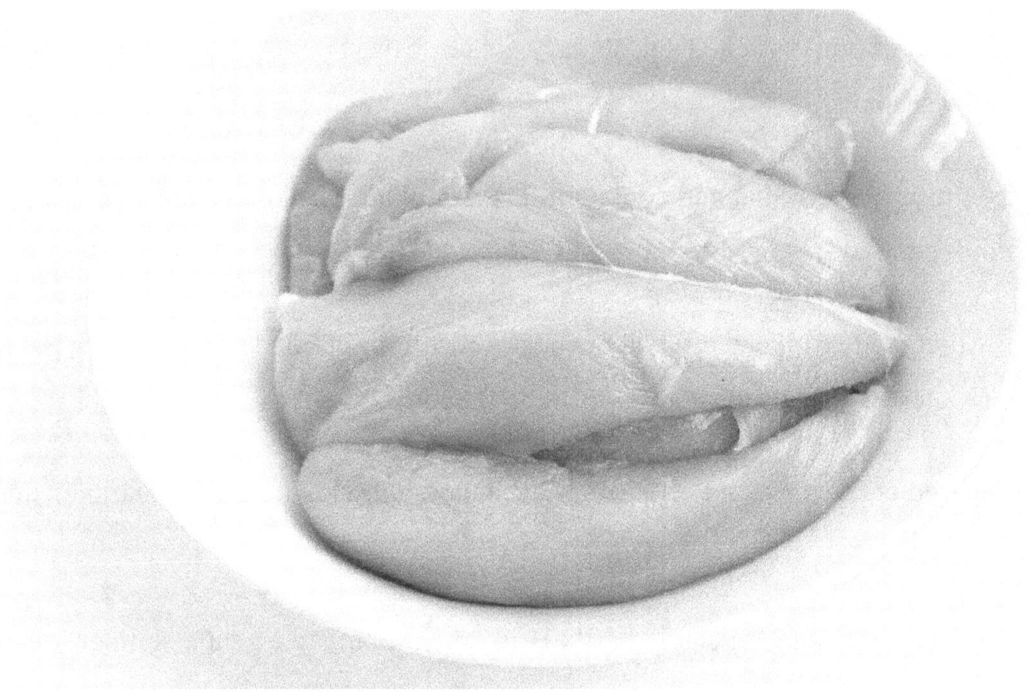

In the realm of gluten-free creations, my Almond-Crusted Baked Chicken Tenders are a delightful revelation. The combination of juicy chicken tenders coated in a crunchy almond crust is a flavor-packed journey that excites the taste buds. As someone who savors the art of crafting wholesome dishes, this recipe holds a special place in my kitchen. Preparing these chicken tenders is like embarking on a culinary adventure—a balance of textures and flavors that make every bite sensational.

Serving Size: 4 servings

Preparation Time: 15 minutes

Cooking Time: 20 minutes

Ingredients:

- Chicken tenders (about 12 tenders)
- Almond flour (1 cup)
- Paprika (1/2 teaspoon)
- Garlic powder (1/2 teaspoon)
- Salt (1/2 teaspoon)
- Cooking spray or olive oil
- Black pepper (1/4 teaspoon)
- Eggs (2)
- Dijon mustard (2 tablespoons)

Instructions:

Preheat your oven to 400°F (200°C) and line a baking sheet with parchment paper. Set up a breading station by placing almond flour in a shallow bowl and whisking eggs and Dijon mustard together in another shallow bowl.

To the almond flour, add paprika, garlic powder, salt, and black pepper. Mix well to evenly distribute the seasonings.

Dip each chicken tender into the egg-Dijon mixture, allowing any excess to drip off. Next, coat the tender with the seasoned almond flour, pressing gently to adhere to the coating.

Arrange the coated chicken tenders on the prepared baking sheet. Make sure to leave some space between them for even cooking.

Lightly spray the chicken tenders with cooking spray or brush them with a thin layer of olive oil. This step helps to achieve a golden and crispy crust. Bake in the preheated oven for about 18-20 minutes, or until the chicken is cooked through and the almond crust is golden.

Remove the Almond-Crusted Baked Chicken Tenders from the oven and let them cool slightly before serving. They're ready to be enjoyed with your favorite dipping sauce.

10. Mediterranean Grilled Eggplant Rolls with Hummus

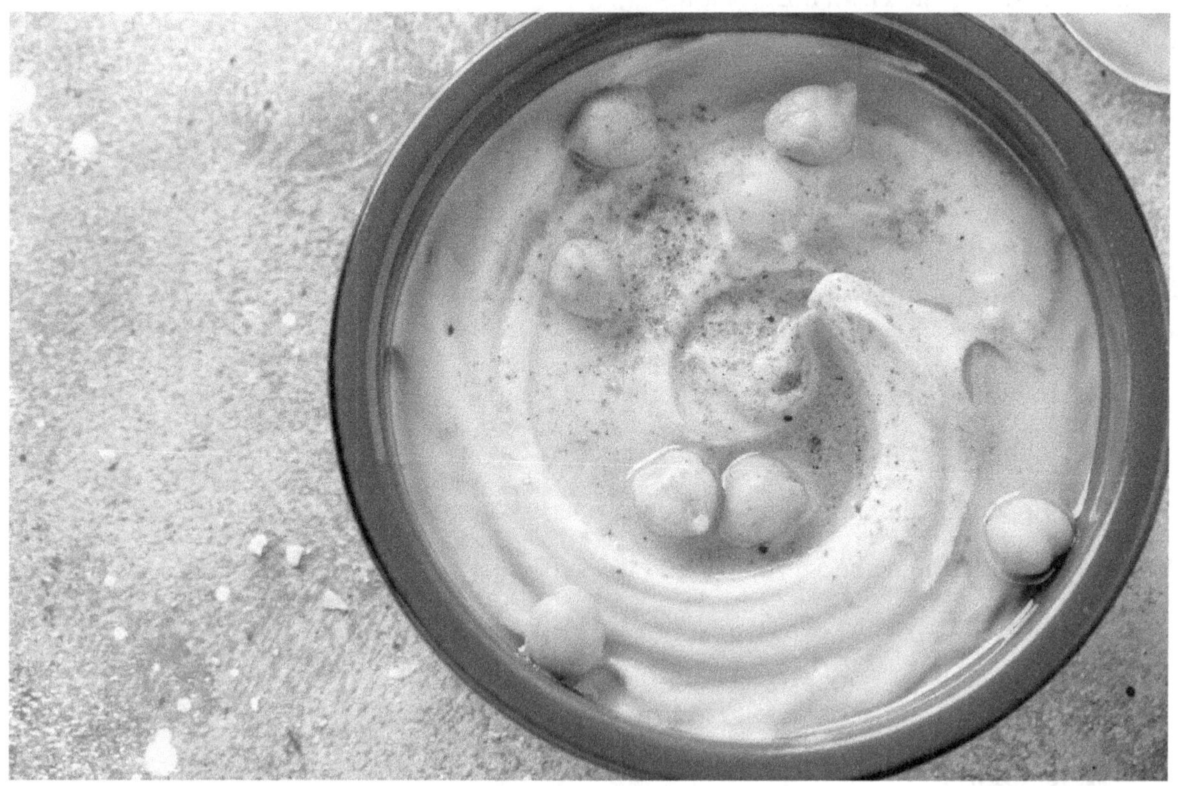

Embarking on a gluten-free culinary adventure, my Mediterranean Grilled Eggplant Rolls with Hummus is a harmonious fusion of flavors that transport me to the sun-kissed shores of the Mediterranean. The marriage of smoky grilled eggplant, velvety hummus, and vibrant herbs is a symphony that dances on the palate. As someone who cherishes the art of crafting elegant appetizers, this recipe holds a special place in my repertoire. Preparing these eggplant rolls is like painting a canvas of taste—an arrangement of ingredients that captures the essence of Mediterranean cuisine.

Serving Size: 4 servings (approximately 12 rolls)

Preparation Time: 20 minutes

Cooking Time: 15 minutes

Ingredients: For the Grilled Eggplant:

- Large eggplant, sliced lengthwise into 1/4-inch thick strips (1)
- Olive oil (2 tablespoons)
- Salt and pepper, to taste

For the Hummus Filling:

- Hummus (store-bought or homemade) (1 cup)
- Chopped fresh parsley (1/4 cup)
- Chopped Kalamata olives (1/4 cup)
- Crumbled feta cheese (optional) (1/4 cup)
- Juice of 1 lemon
- Salt and pepper, to taste

For Assembling:

- Fresh basil leaves, for garnish
- Extra virgin olive oil, for drizzling

Instructions:

First, preheat a grill or grill pan over medium-high heat.

Brush the eggplant slices with olive oil and season with salt and pepper. Then, grill the eggplant slices for about 2-3 minutes on each side, until they are tender and have grill marks. Remove from the grill and set aside.

In a bowl, combine hummus, chopped parsley, chopped Kalamata olives, crumbled feta cheese (if using), lemon juice, salt, and pepper. Mix well to create a flavorful filling.

Lay out the grilled eggplant slices on a clean surface. Spoon a generous amount of the hummus filling onto each slice. Gently roll up the eggplant slices, enclosing the filling.

Place the Mediterranean Grilled Eggplant Rolls on a serving platter. Garnish with fresh basil leaves for an aromatic touch.

Drizzle a bit of extra virgin olive oil over the eggplant rolls. The oil adds a luxurious finish and enhances the flavors.

Your Mediterranean Grilled Eggplant Rolls with Hummus are ready to be savored. The combination of textures and tastes is a testament to the allure of Mediterranean cuisine.

11. Creamy Broccoli and Cheddar Soup

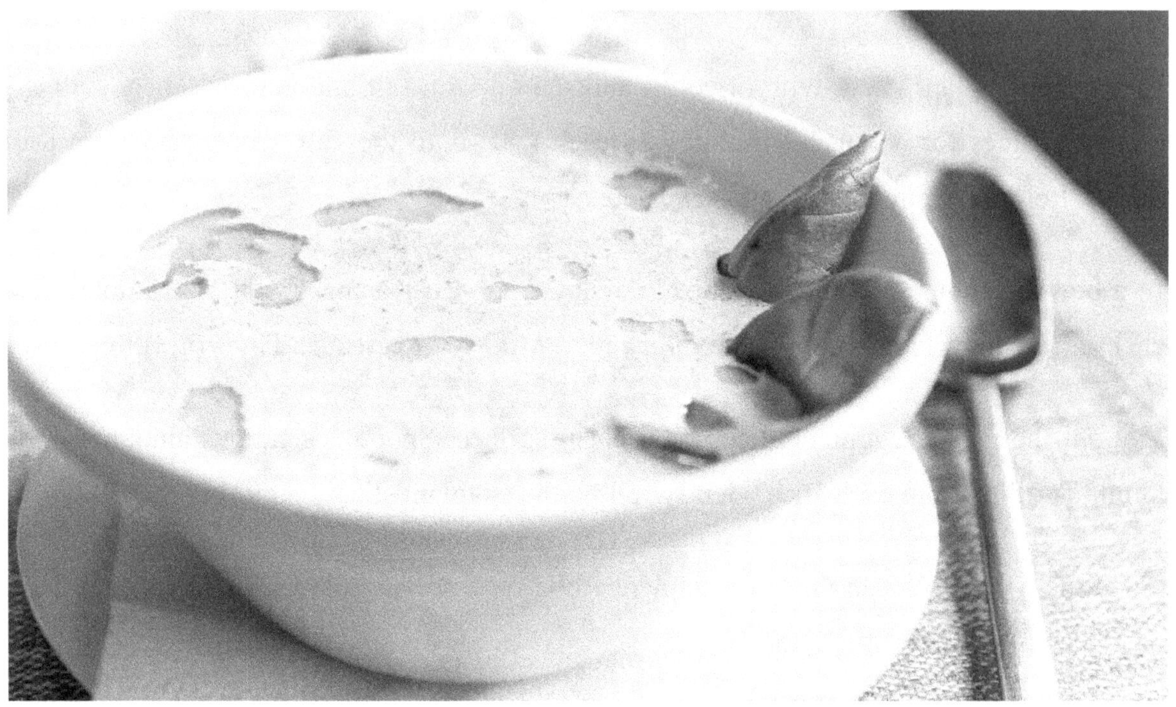

In the realm of gluten-free comfort, my Creamy Broccoli and Cheddar Soup is a warm embrace for the senses. The melding of velvety textures, earthy broccoli, and the rich depth of cheddar is a bowl of pure coziness. As someone who delights in crafting nourishing soups, this recipe holds a special place in my heart. Preparing this soup is like composing a symphony of flavors—a harmony that soothes the soul and warms the spirit.

Serving Size: 4 servings

Preparation Time: 10 minutes

Cooking Time: 25 minutes

Ingredients:

- Butter or olive oil (2 tablespoons)
- Onion, chopped (1)
- Garlic, minced (2 cloves)
- Fresh broccoli florets (3 cups)
- Vegetable or chicken broth (3 cups)
- Milk (dairy or non-dairy) (1 cup)
- Shredded cheddar cheese (1 cup)
- Salt and pepper, to taste
- Optional toppings: extra shredded cheddar, chopped fresh parsley

Instructions:

In a large pot, melt butter or heat olive oil over medium heat. Add chopped onion and sauté for about 2-3 minutes until translucent. Stir in minced garlic and cook for an additional 30 seconds.

Add the fresh broccoli florets to the pot. Sauté for a few minutes until they start to soften slightly.

Pour in the vegetable or chicken broth and milk. Bring the mixture to a gentle simmer.

Allow the soup to simmer for about 15-20 minutes, until the broccoli is tender. Using an immersion blender or regular blender, carefully blend the soup until smooth and creamy.

Return the blended soup to the pot and stir in the shredded cheddar cheese. Allow the cheese to melt and create a lusciously creamy texture.

Season the soup with salt and pepper to taste. Ladle the Creamy Broccoli and Cheddar Soup into bowls.

For an extra touch of indulgence, top the soup with a sprinkle of shredded cheddar cheese and chopped fresh parsley.

12. Herbed Quinoa-Stuffed Bell Peppers

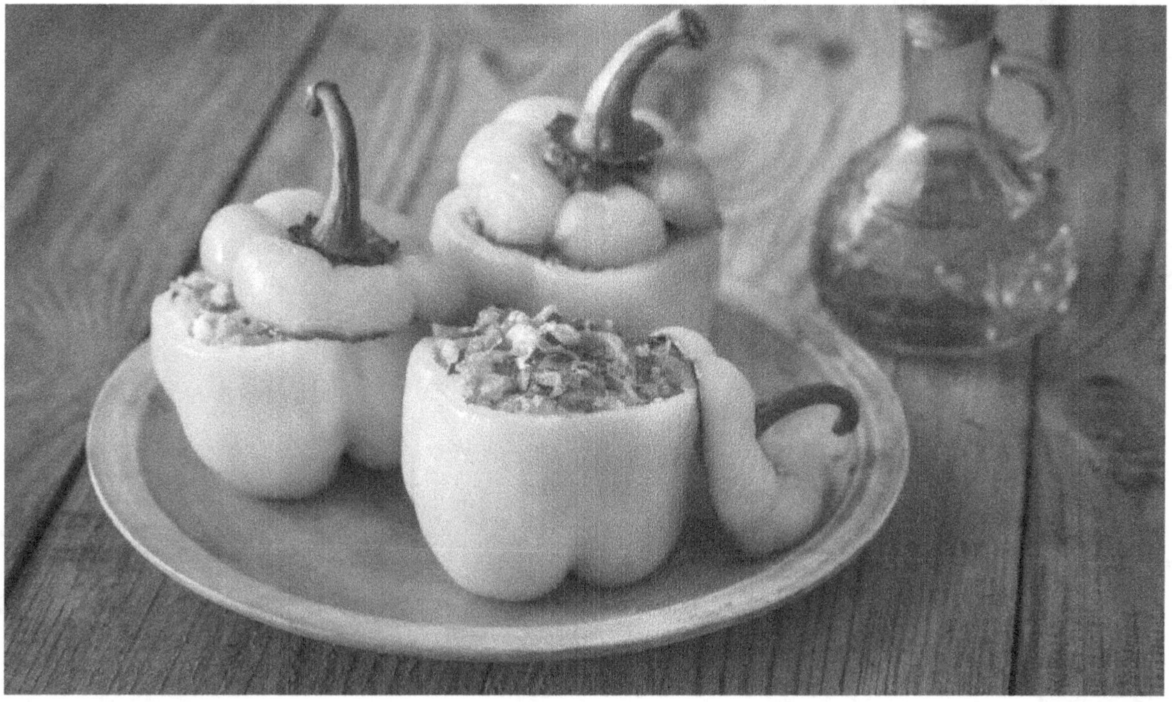

The marriage of fluffy quinoa, aromatic herbs, and the natural sweetness of bell peppers is a symphony of tastes that captivates with every bite. As someone who revels in creating dishes that celebrate the beauty of nature's bounty, this recipe holds a special place in my kitchen. Preparing these stuffed peppers is like weaving a tapestry of taste—a blend of ingredients that harmonize in a sensational medley.

Serving Size: 4 servings (2 halves per serving)

Preparation Time: 20 minutes

Cooking Time: 30 minutes

Ingredients:

- Large bell peppers (red, yellow, or orange) (2)
- Quinoa rinsed and drained (1 cup)
- Vegetable broth or water (2 cups)
- Olive oil (1 tablespoon)
- Small onion, finely chopped (1)
- Garlic, minced (2 cloves)
- Dried thyme (1 teaspoon)
- Dried oregano (1 teaspoon)
- Chopped fresh parsley (1/2 cup)
- Salt and pepper, to taste
- Crumbled feta cheese (optional) (1/2 cup)
- Lemon wedges, for serving

Instructions:

Preheat the oven to 375°F (190°C).

Cut the bell peppers in half lengthwise and then remove the seeds and membranes. Place the pepper halves in a baking dish, cut side up.

In a medium saucepan, combine quinoa and vegetable broth or water. Bring to a boil, then reduce the heat to low and cover. Simmer for about 15 minutes, or until the quinoa is cooked and the liquid is absorbed. Remove from heat and fluff with a fork.

In a skillet, heat olive oil over medium heat. Add chopped onion and sauté until translucent. Stir in minced garlic, dried thyme, and dried oregano, and cook for an additional 1-2 minutes.

In a large bowl, combine the cooked quinoa, sautéed onion mixture, chopped fresh parsley, and crumbled feta cheese (if using). Mix well to distribute the flavors evenly. Season with salt and pepper to taste.

Generously stuff each bell pepper half with the quinoa mixture. Press down gently to pack the filling.

Cover the baking dish with aluminum foil and bake in the preheated oven for about 20 minutes, or until the peppers are tender.

Remove the Herbed Quinoa-Stuffed Bell Peppers from the oven and serve them warm. Squeeze fresh lemon juice over the peppers just before devouring.

13. Gluten-Free Blueberry Muffins with Streusel Topping

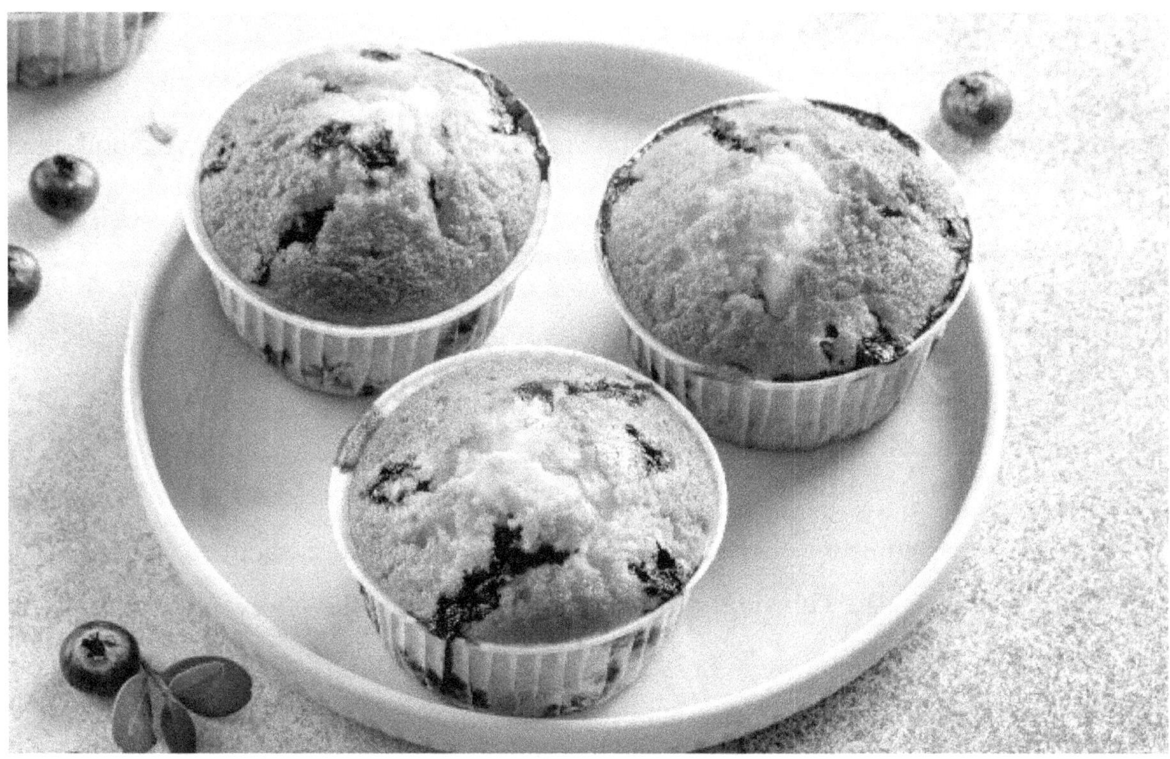

The union of plump blueberries, tender crumbs, and the sweet crunch of streusel is a symphony of textures and flavors that brings joy to gluten-free enthusiasts like me. As someone who embraces the art of gluten-free baking with open arms, this recipe holds a special place in my kitchen. Baking these muffins is like composing a melody of taste—a harmonious blend of ingredients that cater to both the heart and the palate.

Serving Size: 12 muffins

Preparation Time: 15 minutes

Baking Time: 20-25 minutes

Ingredients: For the Muffins:

- Gluten-free all-purpose flour blend (2 cups)
- Baking powder (1 teaspoon)
- Baking soda (1/2 teaspoon)
- Salt (1/4 teaspoon)
- Unsalted butter, melted and cooled (1/2 cup)
- Granulated sugar (3/4 cup)
- Eggs (2)
- Vanilla extract (1 teaspoon)
- Plain Greek yogurt (1 cup)
- Fresh blueberries (1 cup)
- For the Streusel Topping:
- Gluten-free all-purpose flour blend (1/4 cup)
- Granulated sugar (1/4 cup)
- Unsalted butter, cold and cubed (2 tablespoons)

Instructions:

Preheat your oven to 375°F (190°C) and line a muffin tin with paper liners.

In a small bowl, combine the gluten-free all-purpose flour and granulated sugar for the streusel topping. Cut in the cold butter using a fork or your fingers until the mixture resembles coarse crumbs. Set aside.

In a large mixing bowl, whisk together the gluten-free all-purpose flour, baking powder, baking soda, and salt.

In a separate bowl, whisk together the melted butter and granulated sugar until well combined. Add in the eggs and vanilla extract, whisking until the mixture is smooth. Stir in the plain Greek yogurt.

Gradually add the wet ingredients to the dry ingredients and mix until just combined. Be careful not to overmix.

Gently fold the fresh blueberries into the muffin batter.

Divide the batter evenly among the prepared muffin cups, filling each about 2/3 full.

Sprinkle the streusel topping generously over each muffin.

Bake the muffins in the preheated oven for 20-25 minutes, or until a toothpick inserted into the center of a muffin comes out clean.

Allow the muffins to cool in the tin for a few minutes before transferring them to a wire rack to cool completely.

14. Chocolate Avocado Mousse with Berries

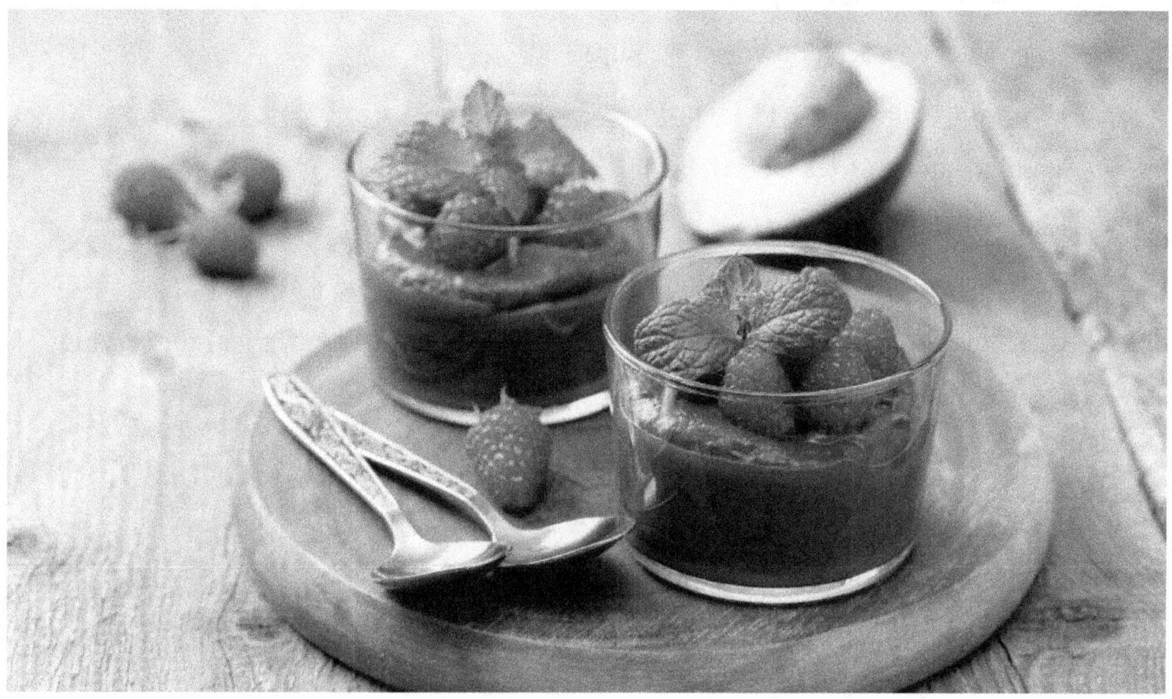

The fusion of luscious avocado, rich cocoa, and the burst of fresh berries is a symphony of flavors that dances on the palate. As someone who delights in crafting desserts that celebrate the marriage of health and decadence, this recipe holds a special place in my kitchen. Preparing this mousse is like painting a canvas of taste—a masterpiece that invites you to savor every spoonful and relish in guilt-free pleasure.

Serving Size: 4 servings

Preparation Time: 15 minutes

Chilling Time: 1-2 hours

Ingredients:

- Avocados, peeled and pitted (2)
- Unsweetened cocoa powder (1/2 cup)
- Honey or maple syrup (1/4 cup)
- Vanilla extract (1 teaspoon)
- Pinch of salt
- Coconut milk or almond milk (1/4 cup)
- Fresh mixed berries (such as strawberries, blueberries, raspberries) for serving
- Optional toppings: shaved dark chocolate, mint leaves

Instructions:

In a food processor or blender, combine the unsweetened cocoa powder, ripe avocados, honey or maple syrup, vanilla extract, and a pinch of salt.

Blend the ingredients until you achieve a creamy and smooth consistency, scraping down the sides of the bowl as needed.

Gradually add the coconut milk or almond milk while continuing to blend. The liquid will help achieve the desired mousse-like texture.

Taste the mousse and adjust the sweetness or cocoa level if desired.

Transfer the chocolate avocado mousse into individual serving bowls or glasses. Cover and refrigerate for at least 1-2 hours to allow the flavors to meld and the mousse to set.

Before serving, top each bowl of mousse with a medley of fresh mixed berries. For an added touch of elegance, garnish with shaved dark chocolate and a few mint leaves.

15. Spaghetti Squash Primavera with Garlic-Herb Sauce

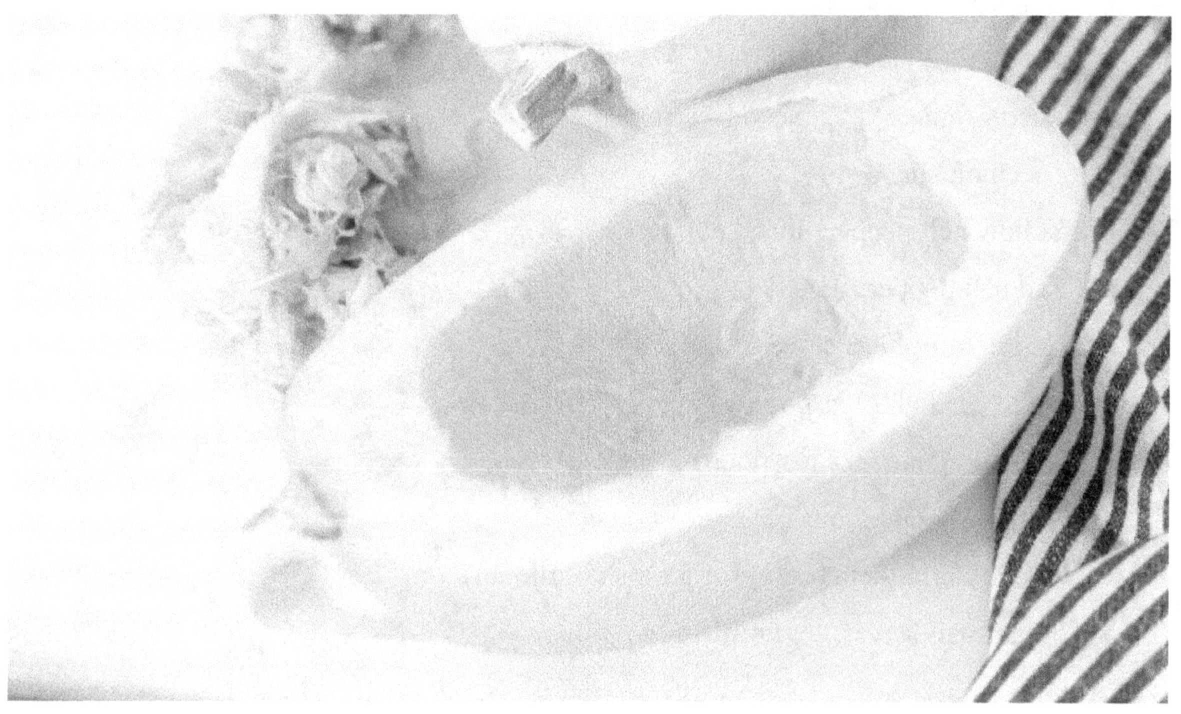

Embarking on a gluten-free culinary journey, my Spaghetti Squash Primavera with Garlic-Herb Sauce is a symphony of colors and flavors that celebrates the essence of fresh ingredients. The marriage of delicate spaghetti squash, vibrant vegetables, and the aromatic dance of garlic and herbs is a tribute to the art of creating meals that are both nourishing and sensational. As someone who revels in the magic of gluten-free cooking, this recipe holds a special place in my heart. Preparing this dish is like weaving a tale of taste—a narrative that intertwines health and indulgence in every forkful.

Serving Size: 4 servings

Preparation Time: 15 minutes

Cooking Time: 40 minutes

Ingredients:

- Spaghetti squash (1)
- Olive oil (2 tablespoons)
- Cherry tomatoes, halved (1 cup)
- Zucchini, sliced (1)
- Yellow bell pepper, sliced (1)
- Red bell pepper, sliced (1)
- Garlic, minced (2 cloves)
- Dried basil (1/2 teaspoon)
- Dried oregano (1/2 teaspoon)
- Salt and pepper, to taste
- Grated Parmesan cheese, for garnish (optional)
- Fresh basil leaves, for garnish

Instructions:

Preheat your oven to 375°F (190°C).

Carefully cut the spaghetti squash in half lengthwise. Scoop out the seeds and strings. Place the halves on a baking sheet, and cut side up.

Drizzle the flesh of the spaghetti squash with olive oil and season with salt and pepper. Roast in the preheated oven for about 35-40 minutes, or until the strands of the squash can be easily separated with a fork.

In a skillet, heat olive oil over medium heat. Add minced garlic and sauté until fragrant. Stir in the dried basil and dried oregano.

Add the sliced cherry tomatoes, zucchini, yellow bell pepper, and red bell pepper to the skillet. Sauté for about 5-7 minutes, or until the vegetables are tender yet still vibrant.

Use a fork to separate the strands of the roasted spaghetti squash. Add the spaghetti squash strands to the skillet with the sautéed vegetables. Toss everything together to combine.

Season the Spaghetti Squash Primavera with salt and pepper to taste. Give it a gentle stir to incorporate the flavors. Divide the Spaghetti Squash Primavera among serving plates. If desired, garnish with grated Parmesan cheese and fresh basil leaves.

16. Roasted Beet and Goat Cheese Salad with Balsamic Glaze

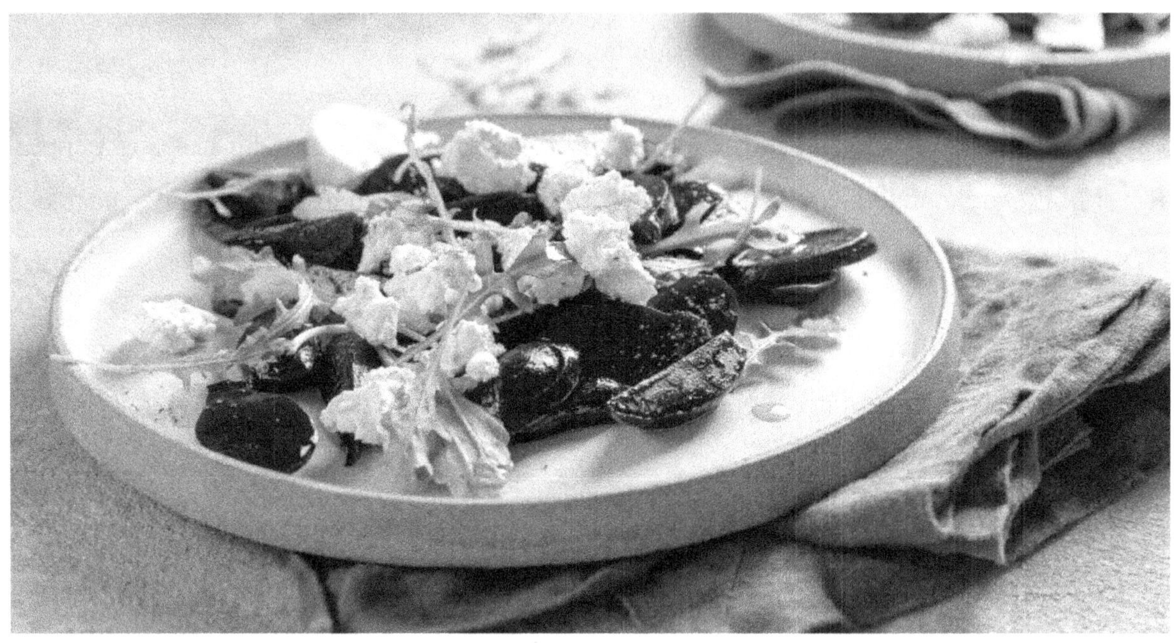

Amidst the realm of gluten-free culinary adventures, my Roasted Beet and Goat Cheese Salad with Balsamic Glaze is a masterpiece of flavors and colors that dance on the plate. The union of earthy roasted beets, creamy goat cheese, and the tangy allure of balsamic glaze is a symphony of contrasts that excites the senses. As someone who embraces the art of gluten-free cooking, this recipe holds a special place in my kitchen. Crafting this salad is like composing a visual and flavorful ode—a poetic creation that celebrates the beauty of vibrant ingredients and the joy of gluten-free living.

Serving Size: 2 servings

Preparation Time: 15 minutes

Cooking and Roasting Time: 45 minutes

Ingredients:

- Medium-sized beets (red, golden, or a mix) (2)
- Mixed salad greens (such as arugula, spinach, or spring mix) (2 cups)
- Crumbled goat cheese (1/4 cup)
- Chopped walnuts or pecans (2 tablespoons)
- Balsamic glaze, for drizzling
- Olive oil (2 tablespoons)
- Salt and pepper, to taste
- Optional garnish: fresh basil leaves

Instructions:

Preheat your oven to 400°F (200°C).

Wash and peel the beets. Cut them into bite-sized cubes.

Place the beet cubes on a baking sheet. Drizzle with olive oil and season with salt and pepper. Toss to coat the beets evenly. Roast in the preheated oven for about 30-35 minutes, or until the beets are tender and slightly caramelized.

In a large bowl, combine the mixed salad greens. Add the roasted beet cubes on top.

Sprinkle the crumbled goat cheese and chopped walnuts or pecans over the salad.

Generously drizzle balsamic glaze over the salad, allowing the flavors to intermingle.

Gently toss the salad to combine all the ingredients without smashing the roasted beets.

Divide the salad among serving plates. If desired, garnish with fresh basil leaves for a touch of aromatic elegance.

17. Oven-baked Garlic Parmesan Fries

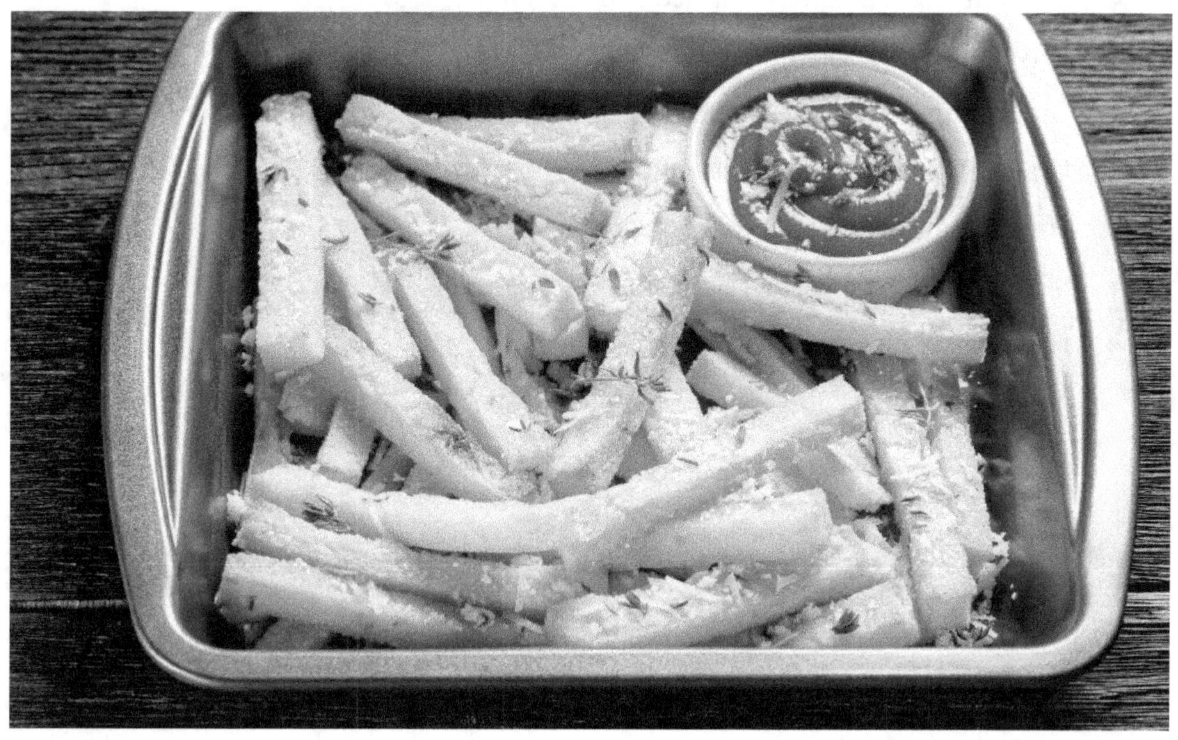

In the world of gluten-free delights, my Oven-Baked Garlic Parmesan Fries are a symphony of flavors and textures that redefine comfort food. The marriage of crispy oven-baked goodness, aromatic garlic, and the savory embrace of Parmesan is a melody that sings to the taste buds. As someone who revels in the art of gluten-free cooking, this recipe holds a special place in my kitchen. Crafting these fries is like a culinary dance—a rhythm of taste that celebrates the joy of indulgence without compromise.

Serving Size: 2-3 servings

Preparation Time: 10 minutes

Baking Time: 25-30 minutes

Ingredients:

- Medium russet potatoes, washed and cut into fries (3)
- Olive oil (2 tablespoons)
- Garlic, minced (2 cloves)
- Grated Parmesan cheese (1/4 cup)
- Dried thyme or rosemary (1 teaspoon)
- Salt and pepper, to taste
- Fresh parsley leaves, chopped, for garnish

Instructions:

First, preheat your oven to 425°F (220°C).

Wash the potatoes thoroughly and cut them into evenly-sized fries. Pat them dry with a clean kitchen towel.

In a large bowl, toss the potato fries with olive oil, making sure each fry is coated.

Add the minced garlic, grated Parmesan cheese, dried thyme or rosemary, salt, and pepper to the bowl. Toss again to evenly distribute the seasonings.

Spread the seasoned potato fries on a baking sheet in a single layer, ensuring they are not overcrowded.

Bake the fries in the preheated oven for 25-30 minutes, flipping them halfway through, until they are golden and crispy.

Once out of the oven, garnish the Oven-Baked Garlic Parmesan Fries with chopped fresh parsley leaves.

Dip your fries in your favorite gluten-free dipping sauce or enjoy them as they are—crispy, savory, and utterly sensational.

18. Mexican Cauliflower Rice Bowl with Guacamole and Salsa

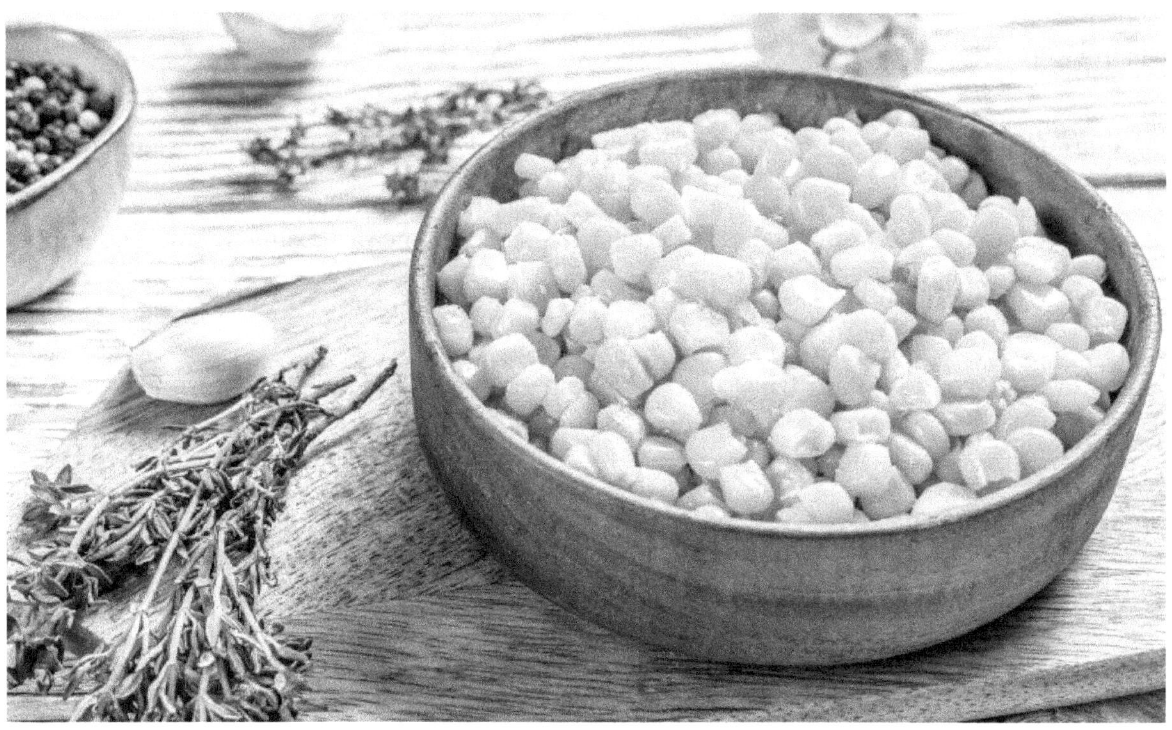

The combo of cauliflower rice, zesty guacamole, and the tangy embrace of salsa is a party for the palate. As a gluten-free enthusiast, this recipe holds a special place in my kitchen. Creating this bowl is like painting a canvas with vibrant hues of taste—a celebration of gluten-free delights that embrace the essence of a Mexican fiesta.

Serving Size: 2 servings

Preparation Time: 15 minutes Cauliflower Rice

Cooking Time: 10 minutes

Ingredients:

- Medium head cauliflower, grated or processed into rice (1)
- Olive oil (1 tablespoon)
- Ground cumin (1 teaspoon)
- Smoked paprika (1 teaspoon)
- Salt and pepper, to taste
- Black beans, cooked and drained (1 cup)
- Corn kernels (fresh, frozen, or canned) (1 cup)
- Diced tomatoes (1 cup)
- Ripe avocado peeled and diced (1)
- Juice of 1 lime
- Chopped fresh cilantro (2 tablespoons)
- Salsa, for serving

Instructions:

Grate the cauliflower or process it in a food processor until it resembles rice-like grains.

In a large skillet, heat the olive oil over medium heat. Add the cauliflower rice, ground cumin, smoked paprika, salt, and pepper. Sauté for about 7-10 minutes, or until the cauliflower rice is tender.

Divide the cooked cauliflower rice between two serving bowls.

Top the cauliflower rice with cooked black beans, corn kernels, and diced tomatoes.

In a separate bowl, mash the avocado with lime juice and chopped cilantro. Season with salt to taste.

Dollop the fresh guacamole onto the cauliflower rice and vegetable layers.

Drizzle your favorite salsa over the bowl for that signature Mexican kick.

Give everything a gentle mix to combine the flavors and textures. Each bite is a dance of tastes that celebrates the essence of Mexican cuisine.

19. Apple Cinnamon Quinoa Porridge

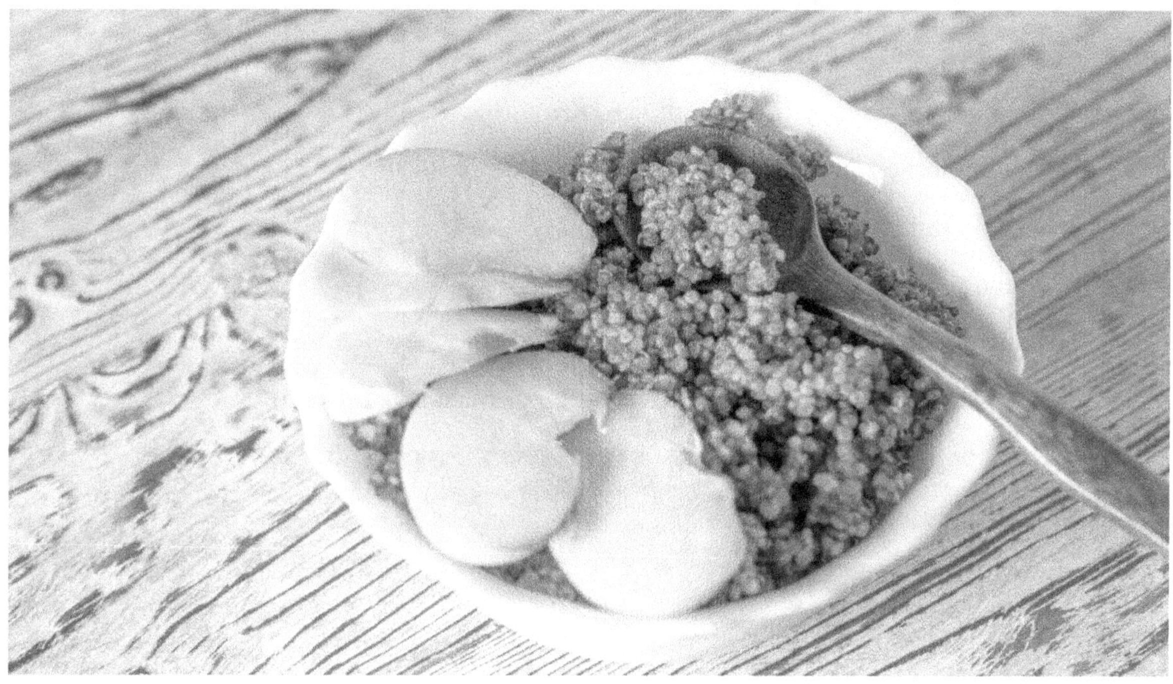

Mornings are a blank canvas for culinary creativity, and one of my favorite ways to infuse comfort and nourishment into my day is with a steaming bowl of Apple Cinnamon Quinoa Porridge. This gluten-free recipe is a symphony of wholesome flavors, combining the nuttiness of quinoa, the sweetness of apples, and the warmth of cinnamon. It's a breakfast that wraps me in a cozy embrace and fuels me with energy for the day ahead.

Serving Size: 2 servings

Preparation Time: 20 minutes

Ingredients:

- Quinoa rinsed and drained (1 cup)
- Water (2 cups)
- Almond milk (or any milk of choice) (1 cup)
- Medium apples, peeled, cored, and chopped (2)
- Ground cinnamon (1 teaspoon)
- Ground nutmeg (optional) (1/4 teaspoon)
- Honey or maple syrup (2 tablespoons)
- Chopped nuts (such as almonds, walnuts, or pecans) (1/4 cup)
- Fresh apple slices and a sprinkle of cinnamon, for garnish

Instructions:

In a medium saucepan, combine the rinsed quinoa and water. Bring to a boil, then reduce the heat to low, cover the saucepan, and simmer for about 15 minutes or until the quinoa is cooked and the water is absorbed. Fluff the quinoa with a fork.

To the cooked quinoa, add the chopped apples, ground cinnamon, and ground nutmeg (if using). Stir well to combine, allowing the flavors to meld and the apples to soften slightly.

Pour the almond milk (or your choice of milk) into the quinoa mixture. Stir gently to combine and achieve your desired porridge consistency. The almond milk adds creaminess and enhances the flavors.

Drizzle in honey or maple syrup and stir to sweeten the porridge to your liking. Adjust the sweetness according to your taste preferences.

In a small skillet over medium heat, toast the chopped nuts until they become fragrant and slightly golden. This step enhances their nuttiness and adds a delightful crunch to the porridge.

Divide the Apple Cinnamon Quinoa Porridge into serving bowls. Top each bowl with a sprinkle of toasted nuts, a few fresh apple slices, and a light dusting of cinnamon.

20. Caprese Salad Skewers with Balsamic Reduction

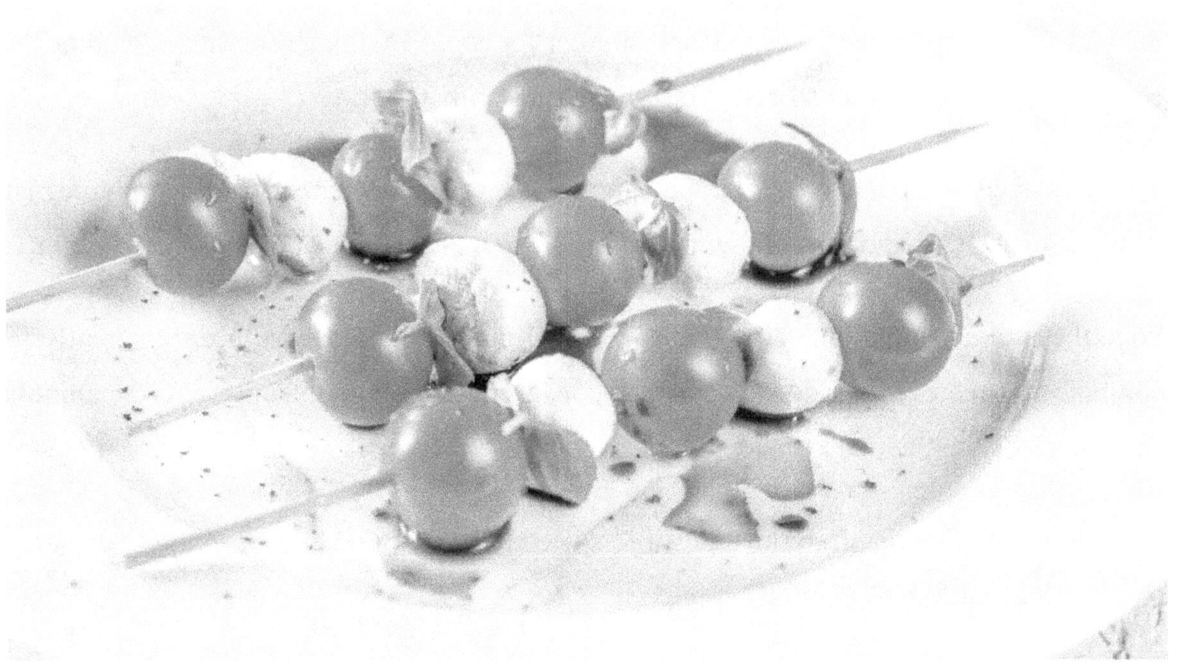

My Caprese Salad Skewers with Balsamic Reduction is a delightful symphony of flavors that transport me to the sun-drenched shores of the Mediterranean. The marriage of juicy tomatoes, creamy mozzarella, and the allure of balsamic reduction is a serenade to the taste buds. As an advocate of gluten-free living, this recipe holds a special place in my kitchen. Crafting these skewers is like weaving a tapestry of taste—a celebration of gluten-free elegance that captures the essence of Mediterranean simplicity.

Serving Size: 4 servings

Preparation Time: 15 minutes

Cooking and Reducing Time: 15 minutes

Ingredients:

- Cherry tomatoes (1 pint)
- Fresh mozzarella balls (8 ounces)
- Fresh basil leaves
- Balsamic reduction, for drizzling
- Olive oil, for drizzling
- Salt and pepper, to taste
- Wooden skewers

Instructions:

Wash the cherry tomatoes and pat them dry. Drain the fresh mozzarella balls. Wash and dry the fresh basil leaves.

Thread a cherry tomato onto a wooden skewer, followed by a fresh mozzarella ball, and then a basil leaf. Repeat the pattern until the skewer is filled.

Place the assembled Caprese salad skewers on a serving platter.

Drizzle balsamic reduction and a touch of olive oil over the skewers, allowing the flavors to intermingle.

Sprinkle a pinch of salt and a grind of black pepper over the skewers to enhance the taste.

Present the Caprese Salad Skewers with Balsamic Reduction with finesse and elegance, embracing the beauty of simplicity.

21. Crispy Baked Fish Tacos with Cabbage Slaw

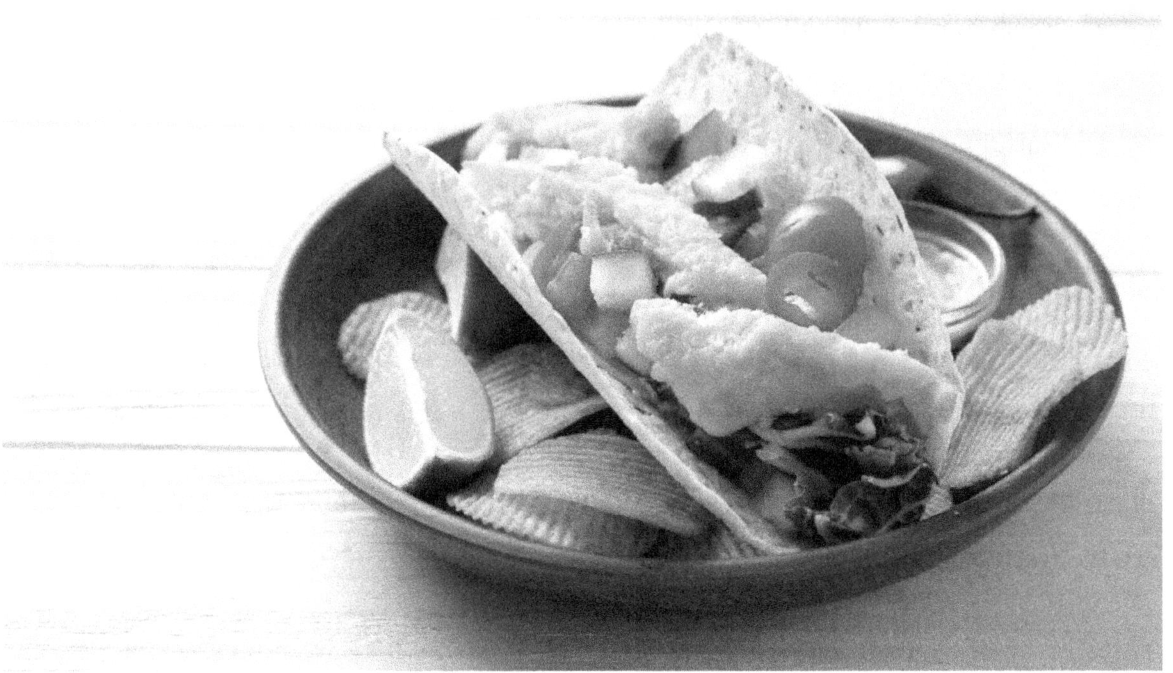

Venturing into the world of gluten-free culinary artistry, my Crispy Baked Fish Tacos with Cabbage Slaw is a symphony of textures and flavors that take me on a journey to coastal retreats. The marriage of golden, crispy fish and the crunch of fresh cabbage slaw is a melody that resonates with my taste buds. As a gluten-free enthusiast, this recipe holds a cherished place in my kitchen. Preparing these tacos is like crafting a canvas of taste—a celebration of gluten-free satisfaction that captures the essence of a seaside escape.

Serving Size: 2-3 servings

Preparation Time: 15 minutes

Baking Time: 15-20 minutes

Ingredients: For the Crispy Baked Fish:

- White fish fillets (such as cod, tilapia, or haddock) (1 pound)
- Gluten-free breadcrumbs (1/2 cup)
- Grated Parmesan cheese (1/4 cup)
- Paprika (1 teaspoon)
- Garlic powder (1/2 teaspoon)
- Salt and pepper, to taste
- Eggs, beaten (2)

For the Cabbage Slaw:

- Shredded green cabbage (2 cups)
- Plain Greek yogurt (1/4 cup)
- Mayonnaise (1 tablespoon)
- Apple cider vinegar (1 tablespoon)
- Honey (1 teaspoon)
- Dijon mustard (1 teaspoon)
- Salt and pepper, to taste

For Assembly:

- Gluten-free corn tortillas
- Fresh cilantro leaves, for garnish
- Lime wedges, for serving

Instructions:

Preheat your oven to 400°F (200°C). Line a baking sheet with parchment paper.

Pat the fish fillets dry with a paper towel. In a shallow bowl, mix the gluten-free breadcrumbs, grated Parmesan cheese, paprika, garlic powder, salt, and pepper.

Dip each fish fillet into the beaten eggs, allowing excess to drip off, and then coat it with the breadcrumb mixture, pressing gently to adhere. Place the coated fillets on the prepared baking sheet.

Bake the fish fillets in the preheated oven for 15-20 minutes, or until they are golden and crispy.

In a bowl, whisk together the Greek yogurt, mayonnaise, apple cider vinegar, honey, Dijon mustard, salt, and pepper. Toss the shredded cabbage in the dressing until well-coated.

Heat the gluten-free corn tortillas according to the package instructions.

Lay a warm tortilla flat, place a crispy baked fish fillet on it, and top with a generous spoonful of the cabbage slaw.

Garnish the tacos with fresh cilantro leaves and serve with lime wedges on the side.

22. Caramelized Onion and Goat Cheese Frittata

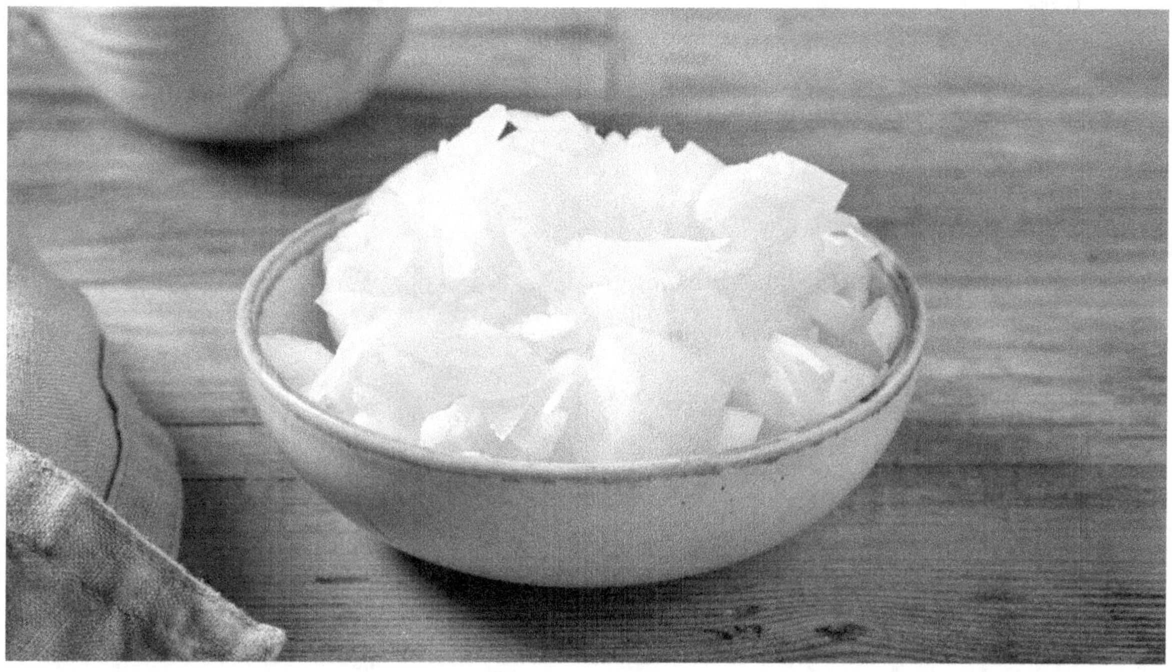

Caramelized Onion and Goat Cheese Frittata is a harmonious symphony of flavors that whisk me away to cozy mornings by the hearth. The dance of sweet caramelized onions and creamy goat cheese creates a melody that serenades my palate. As a dedicated gluten-free aficionado, this recipe holds a treasured place in my kitchen. Crafting this frittata is akin to painting a canvas of taste—a celebration of gluten-free comfort that captures the essence of heartwarming breakfasts.

Serving Size: 4-6 servings

Preparation Time: 15 minutes

Cooking Time: 30 minutes

Ingredients:

- Eggs (8)
- Milk (dairy or non-dairy) (1/4 cup)
- Olive oil (1 tablespoon)
- Onions, thinly sliced (2)
- Salt and pepper, to taste
- Balsamic vinegar (1 teaspoon)
- Crumbled goat cheese (1/2 cup)
- Fresh thyme leaves, for garnish

Instructions:

Preheat your oven to 375°F (190°C).

In a large oven-safe skillet, heat the olive oil over medium-low heat. Add the thinly sliced onions and season with a pinch of salt. Cook the onions, stirring occasionally, until they become soft, golden, and caramelized, about 15-20 minutes. Drizzle balsamic vinegar over the onions and stir to combine.

In a bowl, whisk the eggs and milk together until well combined. Season with a pinch of salt and a grind of black pepper.

Pour the whisked eggs over the caramelized onions in the skillet. Allow the eggs to cook undisturbed for a couple of minutes until the edges begin to set.

Sprinkle the crumbled goat cheese evenly over the frittata.

Transfer the skillet to the preheated oven and bake for 10-15 minutes, or until the frittata is set and slightly golden on top.

Remove the frittata from the oven and let it cool for a few minutes. Garnish with fresh thyme leaves.

23. Pomegranate and Spinach Salad with Honey Mustard Dressing

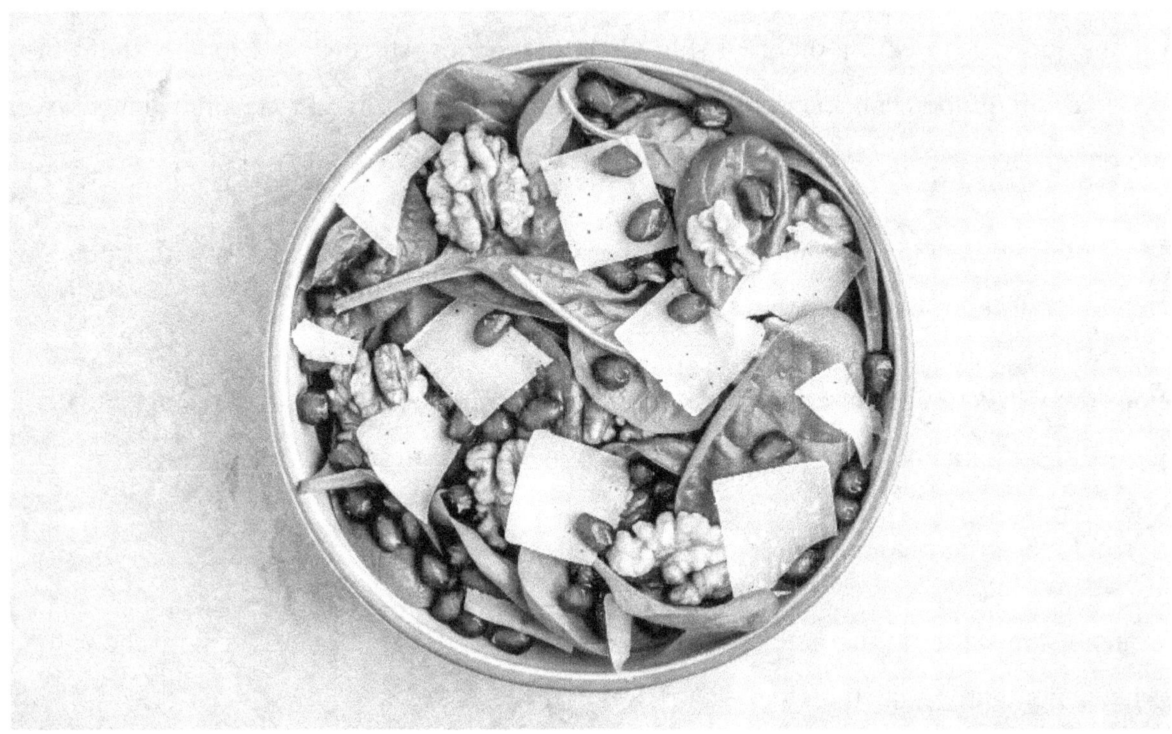

In my gluten-free culinary journey, the Pomegranate and Spinach Salad with Honey Mustard Dressing is a vibrant masterpiece that transports me to a garden of flavors. The union of sweet pomegranate jewels and vibrant spinach leaves dances in my taste buds. As a devoted gluten-free enthusiast, this recipe holds a special place in my heart. Crafting this salad is akin to painting a canvas of taste—a celebration of gluten-free freshness that captures the essence of nature's bounty.

Serving Size: 2-4 servings

Preparation Time: 15 minutes

Ingredients: For the Salad:

- Fresh baby spinach leaves (4 cups)
- Pomegranate arils (1 cup)
- Toasted pine nuts (1/2 cup)
- Crumbled feta cheese (1/4 cup)

For the Honey Mustard Dressing:

- Olive oil (2 tablespoons)
- Apple cider vinegar (1 tablespoon)
- Honey (1 tablespoon)
- Dijon mustard (1 teaspoon)
- Salt and pepper, to taste

Instructions:

In a large salad bowl, combine the fresh baby spinach leaves, pomegranate arils, toasted pine nuts, and crumbled feta cheese.

In a small bowl, whisk together the olive oil, Dijon mustard, apple cider vinegar, honey, salt, and pepper until the dressing is well emulsified.

Drizzle the honey mustard dressing over the salad ingredients.

Gently toss the salad to ensure an even coating of the dressing on all the ingredients.

Divide the salad into serving plates. Sprinkle extra pomegranate arils, pine nuts, and feta cheese on top for a burst of color and flavor.

Each forkful of the Pomegranate and Spinach Salad with Honey Mustard Dressing is an ode to freshness—a medley of textures and a symphony of flavors that encapsulate the essence of gluten-free culinary artistry.

24. Baked Portobello Mushrooms with Quinoa Stuffing

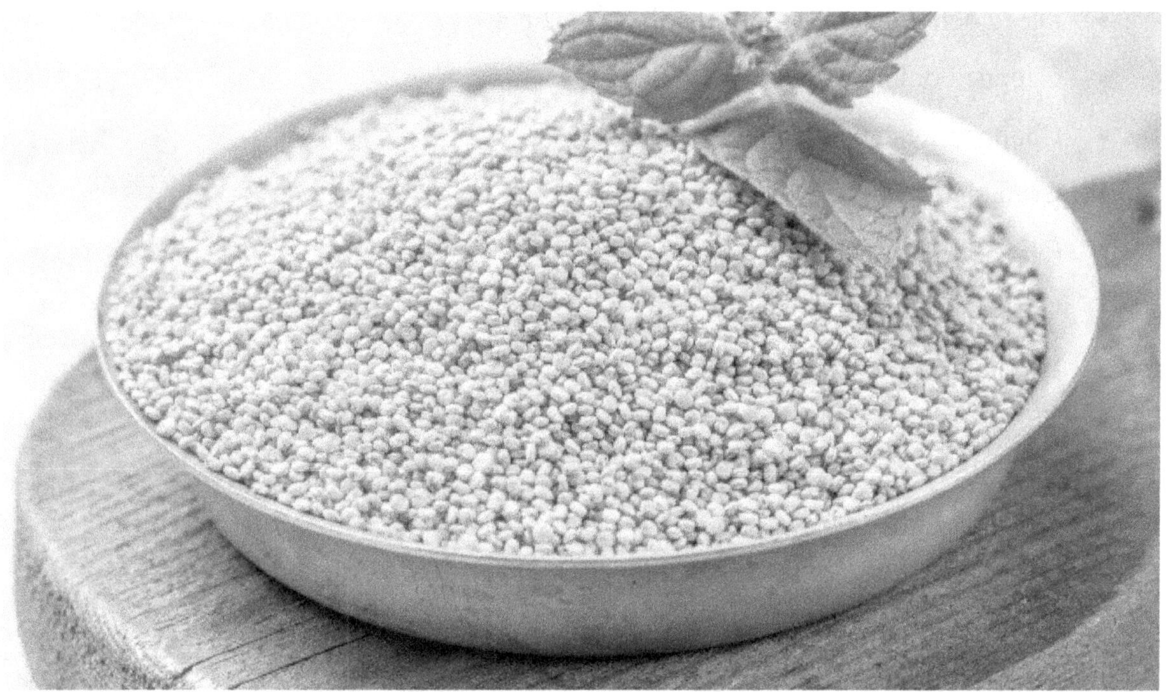

The robust flavors of earthy portobello mushrooms and the nutty embrace of quinoa create a symphony that resonates in each bite. As an ardent gluten-free enthusiast, this dish holds a cherished place in my kitchen repertoire. Preparing this dish is like sculpting a creation of taste—a tribute to gluten-free delight that encapsulates the essence of wholesome satisfaction.

Serving Size: 2-4 servings

Preparation Time: 20 minutes

Cooking Time: 25 minutes

Ingredients:

- Large Portobello mushrooms, stems removed (4)
- Cooked quinoa (1 cup)
- Diced bell peppers (assorted colors) (1/2 cup)
- Chopped onion (1/4 cup)
- Chopped fresh parsley (1/4 cup)
- Crumbled feta cheese (1/4 cup)
- Olive oil (2 tablespoons)
- Garlic, minced (2 cloves)
- Salt and pepper, to taste

Instructions:

Preheat your oven to 375°F (190°C).

Clean the Portobello mushrooms by gently wiping them with a damp cloth. Then, remove the stems and gently scoop out some of the gills to create space for the stuffing.

In a skillet, heat the olive oil over medium heat. Add the chopped onion and diced bell peppers. Sauté until the vegetables are softened.

Add the cooked quinoa to the skillet and mix well with the sautéed vegetables. Stir in the minced garlic and chopped fresh parsley. Season with salt and pepper to taste.

Place the cleaned Portobello mushrooms on a baking sheet. Fill each mushroom cap with a generous portion of the quinoa stuffing.

Transfer the baking sheet to the preheated oven and bake for about 20-25 minutes, or until the mushrooms are tender and the stuffing is heated through.

In the final few minutes of baking, sprinkle crumbled feta cheese over the stuffed mushrooms and allow it to melt slightly.

Remove the Baked Portobello Mushrooms with Quinoa Stuffing from the oven and let them cool for a minute. Serve the mushrooms on a plate, and savor the blend of textures and flavors—a harmony of gluten-free perfection that captivates the senses.

25. Chocolate Peanut Butter Energy Bites

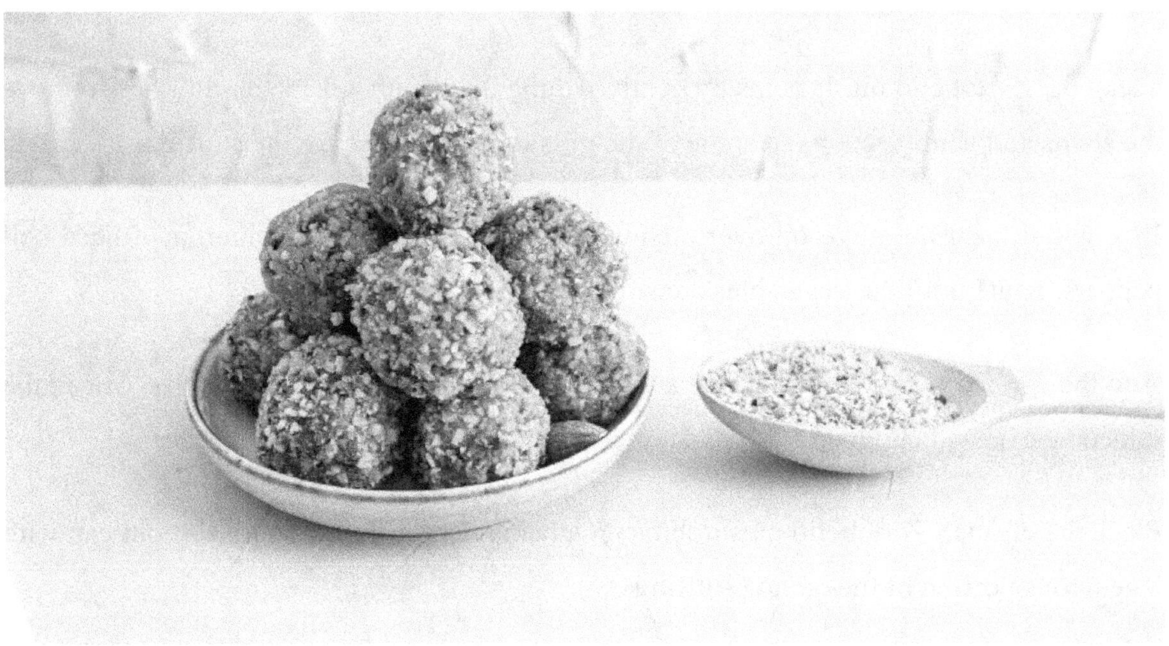

These bites are more than just a snack—they are a burst of energy and a taste of bliss. As a dedicated gluten-free advocate, this recipe holds a special place in my heart. Crafting these bites is like creating a treasure trove of flavor—a celebration of gluten-free goodness that fuels the body and delights the senses.

Serving Size: Approximately 12-15 energy bites

Preparation Time: 15 minutes

Chilling Time: 30 minutes

Ingredients:

- Gluten-free rolled oats (1 cup)
- Creamy peanut butter (1/2 cup)
- Honey or maple syrup (1/3 cup)
- Ground flaxseed (1/2 cup)
- Semi-sweet chocolate chips (1/3 cup)
- Vanilla extract (1 teaspoon)
- A pinch of salt

Instructions:

In a mixing bowl, combine the gluten-free rolled oats, ground flaxseed, creamy honey (or maple syrup), peanut butter, chocolate chips, vanilla extract, and a pinch of salt.

Stir all the ingredients together until they are evenly mixed and form a cohesive mixture.

Using clean hands, take small portions of the mixture and roll them between your palms to form compact energy bites.

Place the formed energy bites on a parchment-lined tray or plate. Chill them in the refrigerator for about 30 minutes. Chilling helps the bites to set and hold their shape.

Once chilled, the Chocolate Peanut Butter Energy Bites are ready to be enjoyed. These bites are a burst of gluten-free goodness—a melody of textures and a celebration of flavors that invigorate and satisfy.

Store any leftover energy bites in an airtight container in the refrigerator. They make for a perfect on-the-go snack or a quick pick-me-up during busy days.

26. Roasted Vegetable Frittata with Fresh Herbs

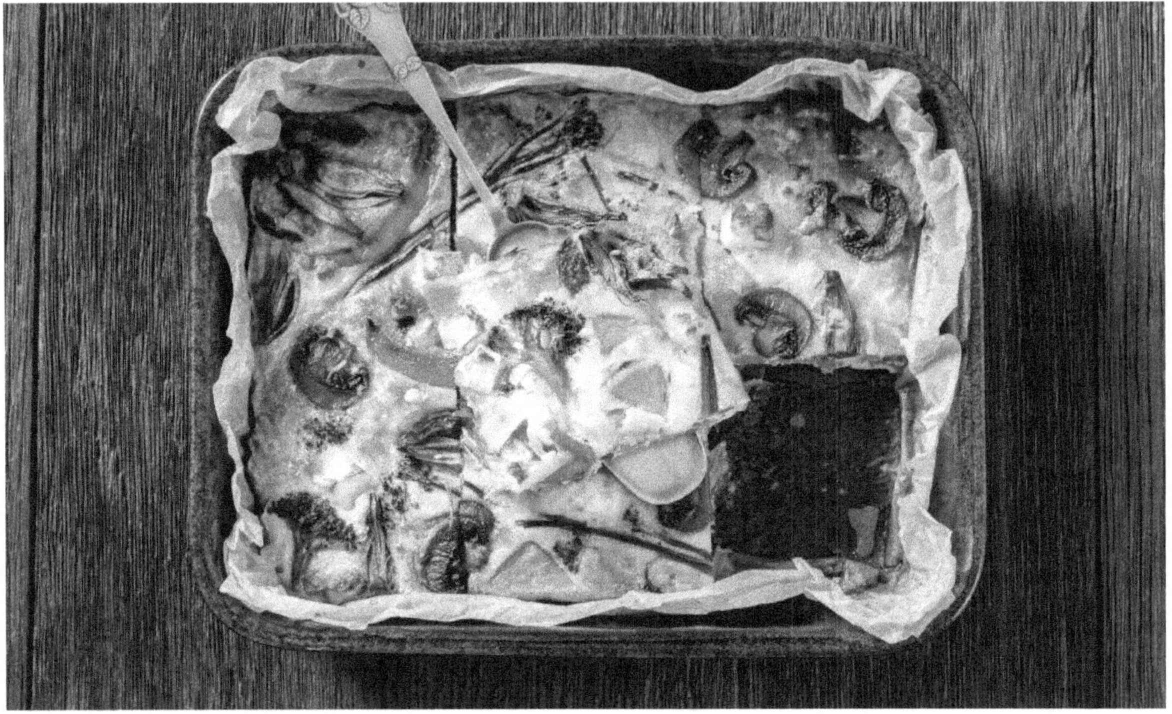

The Roasted Vegetable Frittata with Fresh Herbs holds a cherished place in my heart. This dish embodies the essence of comfort and nourishment, wrapped in a tapestry of vibrant flavors. As a dedicated advocate for gluten-free living, this recipe resonates with my passion for wholesome and delicious meals. Creating this frittata is like painting a canvas of taste—a masterpiece that celebrates the harmony of gluten-free ingredients and culinary creativity.

Serving Size: 4-6 servings

Preparation Time: 15 minutes

Cooking Time: 30 minutes

Ingredients:

- Large eggs (8)
- Milk (dairy or non-dairy) (1/4 cup)
- Assorted roasted vegetables- such as bell peppers, zucchini, and cherry tomatoes (1 cup)
- Chopped fresh herbs- such as parsley, chives, and basil (1/2 cup)
- Salt and pepper, to taste
- Shredded cheese- cheddar, mozzarella, or dairy-free alternative (1/2 cup)
- Olive oil (1 tablespoon)

Instructions:

First, preheat your oven to 375°F (190°C).

In a bowl, whisk the eggs and milk together until well combined. Season with a pinch of salt and pepper.

Heat the olive oil in an oven-safe skillet over medium heat. Add the roasted vegetables to the skillet and sauté briefly to heat them.

Pour the whisked egg mixture over the sautéed vegetables in the skillet. Allow the mixture to cook for a few minutes, gently pushing the edges with a spatula to let the uncooked eggs flow to the sides.

Sprinkle the chopped fresh herbs and shredded cheese evenly over the egg mixture.

Transfer the skillet to the preheated oven and bake for about 15-20 minutes, or until the frittata is set in the center and the cheese is melted and bubbly.

Remove the Roasted Vegetable Frittata with Fresh Herbs from the oven and let it cool slightly. Slice it into wedges and serve warm.

Before serving, garnish the frittata with additional fresh herbs for a burst of color and flavor. Each bite of this frittata is a symphony of taste—a medley of roasted vegetables, fresh herbs, and the comforting embrace of eggs.

27. Blackened Shrimp with Mango-Avocado Salsa

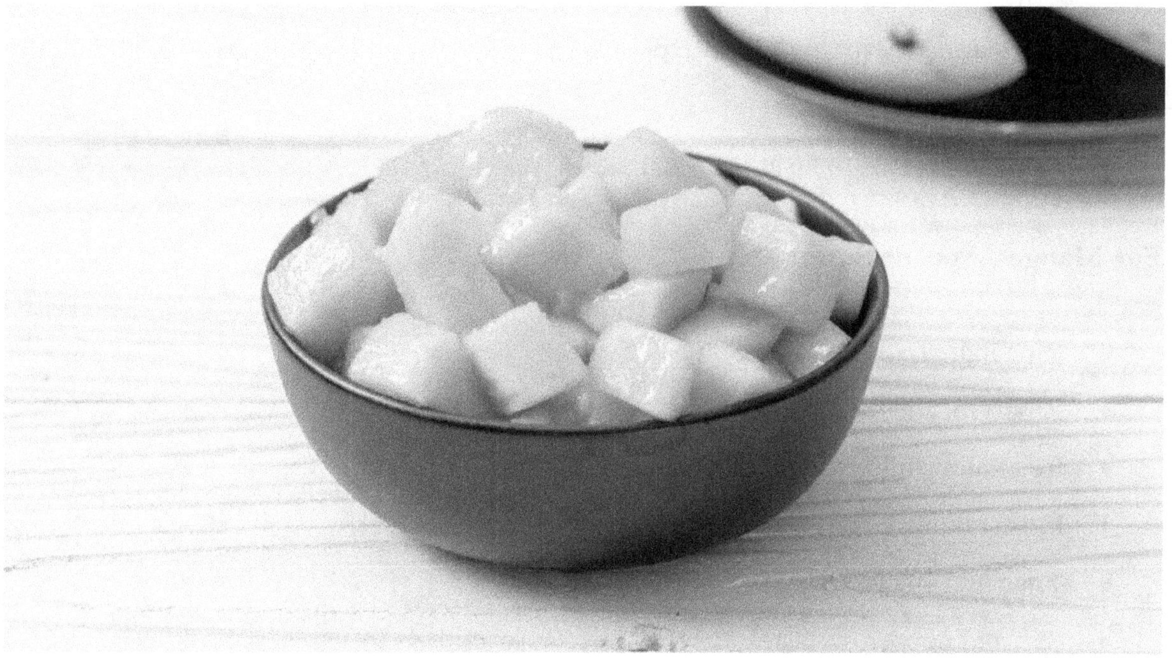

This dish takes me on a journey to tropical shores, where the vibrant colors and bold tastes transport me to a realm of culinary delight. Sharing this recipe is a way of inviting you to experience the harmonious dance of succulent shrimp, zesty blackening spices, and the refreshing embrace of mango and avocado.

Serving Size: 2-3 servings

Preparation Time: 15 minutes

Cooking Time: 10 minutes

Ingredients: For Blackened Shrimp:

- Large shrimp peeled and deveined (1 pound)
- Blackening seasoning (2 tablespoons)
- Olive oil (1 tablespoon)
- Salt and pepper, to taste

For Mango-Avocado Salsa:

- Ripe mango, diced (1)
- Ripe avocado, diced (1)
- Red onion, finely chopped (1/4 cup)
- Fresh cilantro, chopped (1/4 cup)
- Juice of 1 lime
- Salt and pepper, to taste

Instructions:

Pat the shrimp dry with paper towels. In a bowl, toss the shrimp with the blackening seasoning until evenly coated. Season with a pinch of salt and pepper.

Heat the olive oil in a skillet over medium-high heat until it shimmers.

Add the seasoned shrimp to the hot skillet in a single layer. Cook for about 2-3 minutes on each side, or until the shrimp are opaque and cooked through. Remove from heat and set aside.

In a separate bowl, combine the diced mango, chopped red onion, diced avocado, and fresh cilantro. Drizzle the lime juice over the mixture and gently toss to combine. Season with salt and pepper to taste.

Arrange the cooked blackened shrimp on a serving platter. Spoon the mango avocado salsa generously over the shrimp. For an extra touch of elegance, garnish the dish with additional cilantro leaves and a lime wedge.

28. Lemon Poppy Seed Almond Flour Pancakes

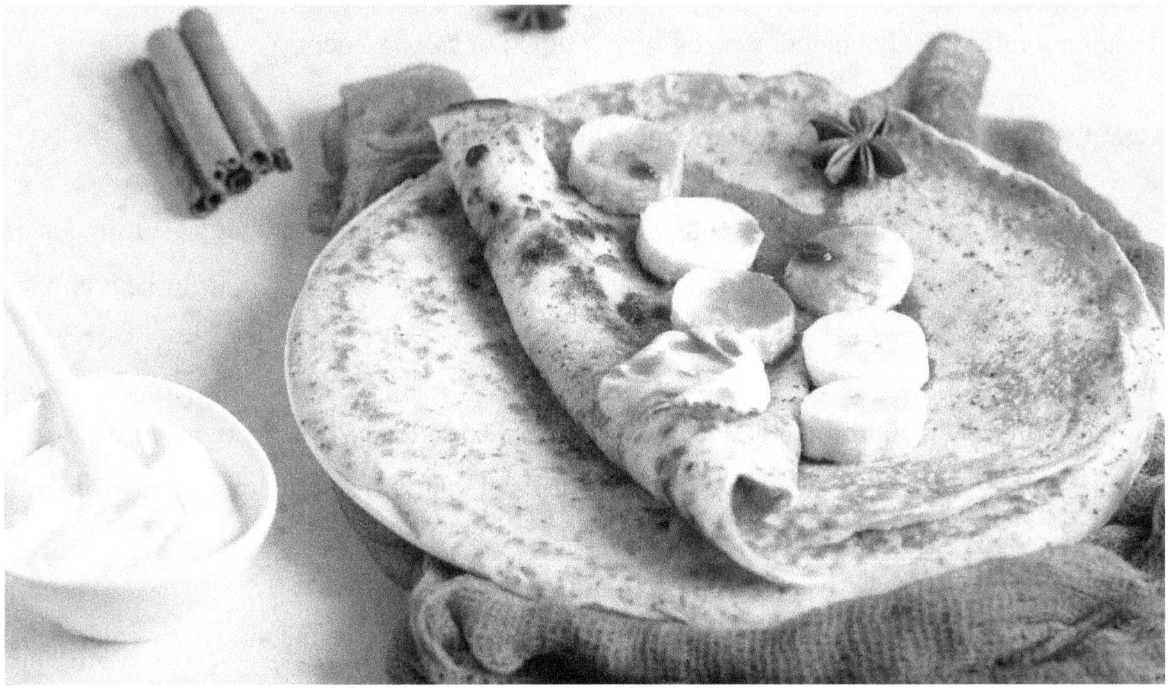

Imagine waking up to a plate of Lemon Poppy Seed Almond Flour Pancakes that effortlessly combine the zesty brightness of lemon with the comforting familiarity of pancakes. These gluten-free wonders are like a burst of sunshine on your plate, filling your kitchen with the delightful aroma of breakfast possibilities. As I mix the batter and watch the pancakes sizzle on the griddle, I'm reminded of how a simple twist on a classic recipe can create something sensational.

Serving Size: 2-3 servings

Preparation Time: 10 minutes

Cooking Time: 15 minutes

Ingredients:

- Almond flour (1 cup)
- Coconut flour (2 tablespoons)
- Poppy seeds (2 tablespoons)
- Baking powder (1 teaspoon)
- Salt (1/4 teaspoon)
- Large eggs (2)
- Almond milk (1/4 cup)
- Zest and juice of 1 lemon
- Honey or maple syrup (2 tablespoons)
- Vanilla extract (1 teaspoon)
- Coconut oil, for cooking
- Fresh berries and maple syrup, for serving

Instructions:

In a mixing bowl, whisk together the almond flour, poppy seeds, baking powder, coconut flour, and salt until well combined.

In a separate bowl, whisk the eggs until slightly frothy. Add the almond milk, lemon zest, lemon juice, honey or maple syrup, and vanilla extract. Mix until the wet ingredients are fully incorporated.

Gradually pour the wet mixture into the dry mixture, stirring gently until just combined. Be careful not to overmix; a few lumps are okay. Let the batter rest for a few minutes to allow the coconut flour to absorb the liquid.

Heat a non-stick skillet or griddle over medium heat. Lightly grease the surface with coconut oil.

Using a 1/4 cup measuring cup, scoop the batter onto the preheated griddle to form pancakes. Use the back of the measuring cup to spread the batter slightly into a round shape.

Sprinkle a few extra poppy seeds onto the surface of each pancake while it's cooking.

Cook the pancakes for about 2-3 minutes on the first side, or until bubbles form on the surface. Flip the pancakes and cook for an additional 1-2 minutes on the other side, until golden brown.

Stack the Lemon Poppy Seed Almond Flour Pancakes on a serving plate. Top with fresh berries and drizzle with maple syrup.

29. Roasted Red Pepper and Tomato Soup

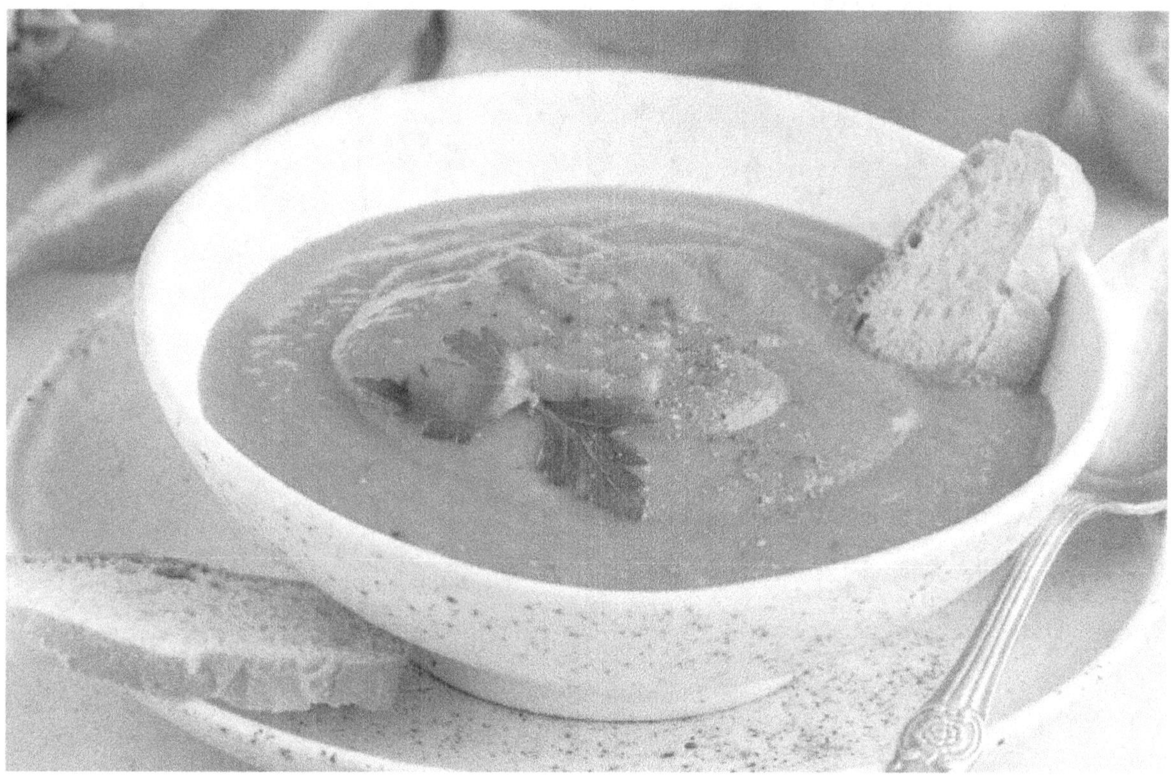

As the weather turns cooler and a comforting meal becomes a necessity, I often find myself craving a bowl of soup that warms both my body and my soul. That's where this Roasted Red Pepper and Tomato Soup comes in. With its vibrant color, rich flavors, and velvety texture, it's like a hug in a bowl. The aroma of roasted vegetables fills my kitchen, and I'm reminded of how food has the power to bring comfort and joy to even the chilliest of days.

Serving Size: 4 servings

Preparation Time: 15 minutes

Cooking Time: 45 minutes

Ingredients:

- Red bell peppers (4)
- Large tomatoes (4)
- Onion, chopped (1)
- Garlic, minced (3 cloves)
- Gluten-free vegetable broth (2 cups)
- Dried basil (1 teaspoon)
- Dried oregano (1/2 teaspoon)
- Red pepper flakes (adjust to taste) (1/4 teaspoon)
- Salt and black pepper, to taste
- Olive oil (2 tablespoons)
- Fresh basil leaves, for garnish
- Dairy-free yogurt or coconut cream, for serving (optional)

Instructions:

Preheat the oven to 400°F (200°C). Cut the red bell peppers in half and remove the seeds. Place the peppers and tomatoes on a baking sheet, cut side down. Roast in the preheated oven for about 25-30 minutes, or until the skins are charred and blistered.

After roasting, remove the peppers from the oven and immediately transfer them to a bowl. Cover the bowl with plastic wrap and let the peppers steam for about 10 minutes. This will make it easier to peel off the skins. Once steamed, carefully peel the skins off the peppers and discard.

In a large pot, heat the olive oil over medium heat. Add the chopped onion and cook until translucent, about 3-4 minutes. Add the minced garlic and cook for another 1 minute, until fragrant.

Add the roasted red peppers, tomatoes, cooked onion, and garlic to a blender. Blend until smooth and creamy. You may need to do this in batches depending on the size of your blender.

Pour the blended mixture back into the pot. Stir in the gluten-free vegetable broth, dried basil, dried oregano, red pepper flakes, salt, and black pepper. Bring the soup to a gentle simmer and cook for about 10-15 minutes, allowing the flavors to meld.

Ladle the Roasted Red Pepper and Tomato Soup into serving bowls. If desired, swirl in a spoonful of dairy-free yogurt or coconut cream for added creaminess. Garnish with fresh basil leaves for a burst of color and an extra layer of flavor.

30. Berry Parfait with Greek Yogurt and Granola

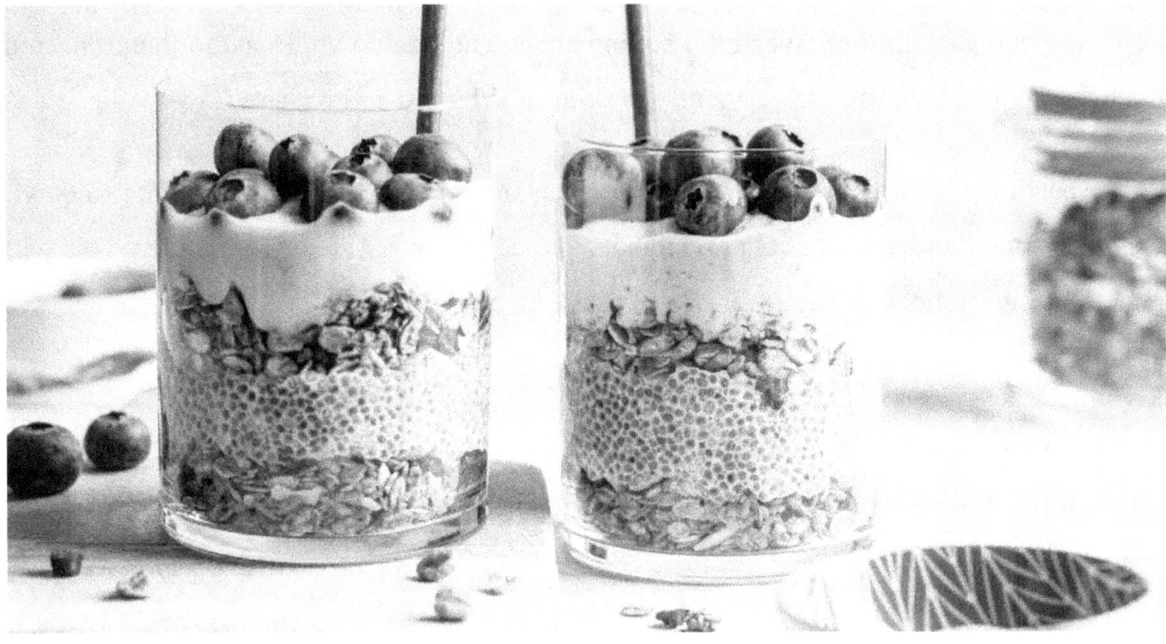

Mornings are a blank canvas, and I often find myself inspired to create a breakfast that's not only nourishing but also a delightful feast for the eyes. That's where this Berry Parfait with Greek Yogurt and Granola comes into play. The vibrant layers of creamy yogurt, ripe berries, and crunchy granola create a symphony of flavors and textures that kick start my day with joy and energy.

Serving Size: 2 servings

Preparation Time: 10 minutes

Ingredients:

- Plain Greek yogurt (dairy-free if preferred) (1 cup)
- Mixed fresh berries- strawberries, blueberries, raspberries, blackberries (1 cup)
- Gluten-free granola (1/2 cup)
- Honey or maple syrup (2 tablespoons)
- Fresh mint leaves, for garnish (optional)

Instructions:

In a bowl, mix the Greek yogurt with a drizzle of honey or maple syrup. Stir well to combine, creating a subtly sweet and creamy base for your parfait.

Rinse the mixed berries under cold water and gently pat them dry with a paper towel. Slice the strawberries into bite-sized pieces, leaving the smaller berries whole for a burst of color and flavor.

In serving glasses or bowls, start by layering a spoonful of the sweetened Greek yogurt at the bottom. Follow with a layer of mixed berries, creating a vibrant mosaic of colors.

Sprinkle a layer of gluten-free granola on top of the berries. The granola adds a delightful crunch and an earthy touch to the parfait.

Repeat the layering process by adding another spoonful of the sweetened yogurt, followed by more mixed berries and granola. You can create as many layers as you like, depending on the size of your serving glasses.

Top the parfait with a final layer of mixed berries, arranging them artfully on the surface. If you have fresh mint leaves on hand, tuck a few leaves between the layers or use them as a charming garnish.

Conclusion

As you turn the final pages of this cookbook, I hope you're inspired and excited to embark on your gluten-free culinary journey. These recipes are more than just meals—they're experiences that showcase the magic of gluten-free cooking.

From the vibrant colors of fresh vegetables to the aromatic medley of herbs and spices, each dish is a reminder that delicious and wholesome go hand in hand. Embrace these gluten-free sensations and discover a world of flavor that will leave you both satisfied and invigorated. Cheers to a delightful adventure in the kitchen!

Appendices

Thank you ♥

Hey, guys! I just wanted to say thanks for supporting me by purchasing one of my e-books. I have to say—when I first started writing cookbooks, I didn't have many expectations for myself because it was never a part of "the plan." It was more of a hobby, something I did for me and decided to put out there if someone might click on my book and buy it because they liked my food. Well, let me just say it's been a while since those days, and it's been a wild journey!

Now, cookbook writing is a huge part of my life, and I'm doing things I love! So, THANK YOU for trusting me with your weekly meal preps, weekend BBQs, 10-minute dinners, and all of your special occasions. If it weren't for you, I wouldn't be able to concentrate on producing all sorts of delicious recipes, which is why I've decided to reach out and ask for your help. What kind of recipes would you like to see more of? Are you interested in special diets, foods made with kitchen appliances, or just easy recipes on a time-crunch? Your input will help me create books you want to read with recipes you'll actually make! Make sure to let me know, and your suggestions could trigger an idea for my next book…

Take care!

Owen